How to obtain fast, drug-free relief from headache

In the same series
ALLERGY HANDBOOK
BANISH BACK PAIN
ECZEMA RELIEF
HAY FEVER HANDBOOK
LOWER YOUR BLOOD PRESSURE

BANISH HEADACHES

A DOCTOR'S PLAN FOR RELIEF WITHOUT DRUGS

Dr Mike Whiteside

THORSONS PUBLISHING GROUP

First published 1990

British Library Cataloguing in Publication Data

Whiteside, Mike
  Banish headaches.
  1. Man. Head. Headaches. Self-treatment
  I. Title
  616'.0472

ISBN 0 7225 1930 3

Published by Thorsons Publishers Limited, Wellingborough, Northamptonshire NN8 2RQ, England

Typeset by Harper Phototypesetters Limited, Northampton, England
Printed in Great Britain by Mackays of Chatham, Kent

10 9 8 7 6 5 4 3 2

Contents

Introduction

For many people, headaches destroy the quality of life and are a social nightmare. The searing pain behind the eye, the crushing sensation on top of the head or the tight band around the forehead can strike at any time. Around 95 per cent of the population suffer from them, with men and women affected equally. Often they are merely a nuisance brought on by overwork, tiredness, stress, or alcohol, but they are still severe enough to send one in three people to consult their general practitioners each year. Unfortunately, doctors usually prescribe painkillers which only suppress the headache without looking at the underlying reason for it. Whilst it is reasonable to take an occasional tablet to relieve them, there is increasing evidence that 'popping' too many aspirin or paracetamol can actually increase the frequency of headaches to the extent that they occur every day. As well as this, aspirin can cause bleeding of the stomach lining, and too much paracetamol can damage the liver. It is the aim of this book, therefore, to look at the underlying situations that can produce headaches and recommend simple, practical, effective methods of dealing with them without resorting to drug therapy. It includes two easy-to-follow charts which can be used for quick reference.

Headaches are frustrating as they frequently occur at socially inconvenient times, e.g. before a dinner party, when it is impossible to rest and relax. Not only that, for some reason it is a condition that evokes little or no sympathy from one's life partner! The same stimuli do not always produce the headaches, so the cause may be difficult to identify. The reason for this is that the body has its own defence mechanism called the immune system to enable it to fight off untoward conditions. If the immune system is in a poor or depressed state then the body is more susceptible to ill-health, and headaches can occur. If it is in tip-top shape then the headaches do not start.

It is important, therefore, to look not only for any obvious causes, but also the factors present which may be lowering the body's defences. These can be lack of sleep, insufficient relaxation, poor exercise pattern, a high stress level, or a deficient diet. Headaches are an end result of these interactions and can be relieved by identifying them and taking the appropriate action.

Around 80 per cent of all headaches arise because of a problem in the person's lifestyle. Only 20 per cent are symptoms of an actual medical condition, of which the commonest are migraine, sinusitis, and high blood pressure. Even these may have been precipitated by some external influence at work or at home. Before writing this book I carried out a survey of over a thousand patients at my surgery who suffered from headaches. Without exception they gave various extrinsic factors not necessarily as the main cause but certainly as playing a major role. By far and away the commonest of these was a smoke-filled room. About one-third of the population of Britain smoke cigarettes, and it is interesting to note that the latest research indicates that there is a greatly increased chance of lung cancer and heart disease in 'passive' smokers compared to those who live and work in a clear environment. Thus, not only does a smoky atmosphere subject us to headaches but it may also put our lives in danger. If you are subjected to this at work then it is vital to ask your employer to deal with the problem. I can only hope that in the near future as many public places as possible will become completely smoke-free. There are encouraging signs now, but my own pet hate is restaurants, which often have no restrictions. There is nothing worse than trying to relax and eat a special meal only to find clouds of smoke drifting over you.

Many patients mentioned a stuffy environment as a cause of headaches. Central heating without adequate ventilation will produce this type of atmosphere and it is important to open windows wherever possible. The other way to counteract it is to use an ionizer which discharges negative ions into the room. This has the effect of producing very clear air and headaches will not develop. Air conditioning has the same effect as central heating in that it removes the negative ions from the atmosphere, and the ionizer will correct this in a similar manner. Other factors at work include artificial light and prolonged use of VDU screens, so obviously sufficient breaks away from these should be included when possible.

In 1890 the book *Virtue's Household Physician* listed the cause of headaches as rich fried foods, working in poor light, eye strain, stimulants including coffee and tea, stress, and sleeping in a hot or badly-ventilated room. It is evident that little has changed in the past hundred years, as these causes are remarkably similar to those of modern times.

All headache sufferers should look for the factors that produce their headaches, but it is often not as simple as it sounds to identify them. To make this easier, it is necessary initially to classify the headaches into certain types, as these usually have the same or similar causes. The first chapter of this book outlines the way to do this, and later chapters explain the methods of curing them. While it is often possible to cure headaches without professional help, this may be needed in the more severe cases. As conventional treatment has only drug therapy to offer with all the associated side-effects, this book explains several types of alternative medical therapy including acupuncture, hypnosis, homoeopathy and osteopathy and how they apply to each particular case. These all have in common the idea that people must be treated as whole individuals with a body, mind and spirit.

Above all, this book has been designed to be practical, and for this reason it is illustrated with case histories based on actual patients and their experiences. Certain details have of course been changed to preserve their identity.

Identification of your headache

CHAPTER 1

Types of headache

Muscular (tension) headaches

Nearly everyone has suffered from this type of headache, and it accounts for four out of five of all those seen in the surgery. These headaches are extremely common and many people experience them every day. The pain is produced by contraction of the muscles of the scalp, and starts at the base of the neck, spreading over the top of the head, and on to the forehead. This classically produces the sensation of a heavy weight pressing down on the head or of a tight band constricting it. Sometimes not all of the scalp muscles are involved and so the pain may be localized to the area where the muscles have tightened. This commonly occurs just above the eyes.

Stress is the usual cause of muscular headaches, though by no means the only one, and for this reason it is a little unfair to blanket them all under the term 'tension'. Anything that causes strain on the muscles of the neck or scalp can trigger the headaches and can simply be from tiredness, unhealthy working conditions, or a poor posture. The latter is usually from staying in the same position for a prolonged period of time. Computer programmers and secretaries are particularly susceptible as they often have to work in an uncomfortable chair, hunched over a keyboard for hours on end. Sitting crouched over the steering wheel on a badly designed car seat on a long journey is a situation common to many of us, with the inevitable muscular headache when we arrive at our destination.

Howard A. was a 41-year-old teacher who came into my surgery one morning complaining that he had developed severe headaches over a period of three months. He described them as similar to someone holding his head in a vice and slowly tightening it. At other times it felt as if the whole world was pressing down on the top of his head. He had tried taking paracetamol with no effect, and had become worried that there might be a serious underlying cause. I was able to reassure him that his physical examination was completely normal, and it was apparent from his description that the headaches were muscular in origin. On closer questioning it turned out they had started at a time when one of the teachers at school had gone into hospital and Howard had doubled up on some of his lessons. This meant that he lost all his free periods, when normally he had time to relax and gather his thoughts together. This lack of available time at school meant he was having to take extra work home to prepare for the following day.

At about the same time, Howard's mother had come to stay until her new bungalow was completed. While usually his relations with his mother were reasonably satisfactory, having her living under the same roof was a totally different matter! I explained to Howard that with all this extra pressure and stress it was not surprising his body should show the strain in some way, and in his case it produced tension headaches. He could see this quite clearly after our discussion and happily, after the teacher recovered and his mother moved, his headaches disappeared.

Howard's was a reasonably simple case to sort out as the causes of the stress, which in turn produced the headaches, were quite obvious. This, however, is not always the position. Sarah B. was a 37-year-old woman with a nine-month history of non-specific headaches which could occur at the back of the head near the neck, on top or even on the forehead above the eyes. They could last for hours, days, or weeks, yet did not seem to have any underlying precipitating cause. She did have a stressful job as a sales representative, but was very successful and enjoyed an excellent standard of living. Again full clinical examination was normal, and although they did not fit the classical textbook description of tension headaches, I was certain that muscular spasm was indeed the underlying problem.

I enquired deeper into Sarah's lifestyle to try to identify the triggering factors. She did have an extremely busy job which frequently involved irregular hours, often working well into the evening. A substantial amount of this time involved selling on the telephone where she was confined in a stuffy office. Her diet was of poor quality, with lunch usually consisting of a sandwich brought in by one of her colleagues from the pub across the road. She had an hour to travel by train in the morning and rarely had time for any breakfast. To meet her sales targets Sarah often took work home at weekends: she had very little time for relaxation and exercise was virtually non-existent. Before cooking her evening meal she would have a large measure of gin and tonic and a couple of cigarettes. This alcohol intake coupled with a rather fatty diet had made her markedly overweight.

There was no doubt in my mind that this quintet of obesity, poor diet, lack of exercise, too much alcohol, and very little relaxation was the cause of her persistent headaches. Each one individually was probably not sufficient to produce them but collectively they were lowering her body resistance to such an extent that the headaches occurred. I explained all this to Sarah who initially found my reasoning hard to accept as originally she had only come to the surgery with the thought that she would be given a few painkillers.

I must have managed to convince her, as three months later she told me she was now walking the mile to the tube station in the morning and had made several other changes to her lifestyle. She was eating a healthier diet with little fat and had lost over a stone in weight. Added to that she had taken up cycling at weekends, which was a hobby she had always enjoyed when a teenager and which she found excellent as a positive form of relaxation. Not surprisingly, the headaches had disappeared and I am certain that, if she maintains this improved lifestyle, they will not recur.

These two cases show that tension headaches can arise from the simple pressures that many people are subjected to every day. In both Howard's and Sarah's cases the reasons for the extra strain were easily remedied, but this may not always be possible. It is often difficult to change working conditions, and emotional stress from family or financial difficulties may be equally impossible to relieve. However, it is simple to modify our reactions to stress, and these alterations invariably lead to elimination of the headaches. This will be discussed in detail in later chapters.

Migraine

I was recently shown a set of pictures painted by migraine sufferers, portraying how they felt during an attack, and it struck me how each demonstrated a very personal view of pain. Each picture was very individual, as is each episode of migraine, although there are nearly always several common features. Migraine is a particularly severe form of headache and can be very debilitating as it is frequently associated with vomiting, diarrhoea, visual disturbances and dizziness. The pain is usually one-sided and is likened to 'being drilled through the side of the head'.

The pain of migraine is caused by a widening of the blood vessels in the lower part of the brain, which brings about the characteristic throbbing headache. Strangely this is often, though not always, preceded by a narrowing of the same arteries which typically produces visual problems before the actual headache. It is thought that these changes arise from the formation of certain chemicals in the brain stem, the production of which is stimulated by external factors. Similarly to muscular headaches, stress is the most important precipitating factor, although there are several others, as illustrated in the cases below.

Mike B. was a 39-year-old insurance salesman who came into my consulting room with a look of intense fear on his face. His work involved visiting people at their homes by appointment and selling policies to them. The day before, a friend had asked him to play a squash match at lunch-time and Mike agreed, as he was keen to improve his fitness. Unfortunately, on the morning of the game his first client kept him talking considerably longer than arranged, and from then on he was rushing round trying to make up lost time. He just made it to the leisure centre where he was playing, but was hardly in a relaxed frame of mind. After ten minutes he became aware of the sensation of flashing lights in his right eye. Soon after, he noticed that at certain points on the court he was unable to actually see the squash ball. Mike was most alarmed by this but managed to finish the game, though he was soundly beaten. After a relaxing hot shower his vision returned to normal and he was able to continue his work.

Midway through the afternoon he developed a right-sided headache of such severity that he had to cancel his remaining engagements and return home. His eyes had become very sensitive to light and he retired to bed with the curtains closed. Whilst he had occasionally suffered from tension headaches in the past, Mike had never experienced anything as severe as this and the pain seemed to bore right through his head. Over the subsequent few hours he developed profuse vomiting and it was only when he finally drifted off to sleep that the headaches eased. The next morning when I saw him he was almost back to normal.

His main concern was that with this bizarre story he had developed a brain tumour. Most people with headaches worry about this, but in my eleven years of general practice I have only seen one cancerous growth in the brain. However it is routine to exclude this condition and happily Mike's physical examination was normal. It was clear that he had experienced a classical attack of migraine, which can start at any age. The initial constriction of the blood vessels in the brain had caused his symptoms on the squash court, producing the flashing lights and in Mike's case a loss of part of the field of vision. The next phase, where the arteries widen, may not follow until several hours later and indeed may not occur at all. This dilation creates the headache, sensitivity to light, and vomiting.

This episode of migraine was totally related to stress, and Mike readily admitted that it had been unwise to fit in a highly strenuous game in an already busy day. I think that knowledge will prevent the same sort of circumstances occurring again and it is therefore unlikely he will suffer another attack.

In many the picture is not so clear and consequently they have repeated bouts of migraine which can wreak havoc in their day to day routine. Janet M. was a 28-year-old secretary who had complained of headaches for the past five years. These happened on a regular basis every three to four weeks and were always on the left side of her face just above the eyebrow. She did not have any disturbance of vision or any warning that the headaches were coming on. Fortunately she did not actually vomit with them, but the nausea was intense and most unpleasant. She had found that only by resting in complete silence could she relieve the symptoms. As Janet was usually at work when it happened, this was difficult and did not make her popular with her employers.

This type of migraine was similar to that described in the first case except that the constriction of the blood vessels at the onset of the attack was not severe enough to cause any visual problems.

We looked very closely into her lifestyle for the trigger factors. The onset of the headaches seemed to coincide with her marriage five years ago and it was at that time she started taking the oral contraceptive pill. Janet had wondered at the time whether the headaches were related to the pill, and in fact she had only stayed on it for six months. As the headaches had persisted she had assumed that they were not connected with the pill. There is, however, a strong relationship between the pill and migraine. Rather than actually causing migraine, it may unmask a tendency to develop it, as stopping the pill often does not lead to disappearance of the headaches. It is routine nowadays to advise women not to start on the pill if there is a strong family history of migraine.

As Janet was a secretary she did spend some time in front of a VDU screen and her office was lit with strip-lights. Both of these have been shown to trigger migrainous attacks. So the contraceptive pill and bright lights seemed to be the causative factors in Janet's case. Unfortunately as she had already stopped the pill, and was unable to change her office conditions, there was little she could do about them. Even so, by following the guidance described in the later chapters she was able to virtually eliminate her headaches.

Grace N. was a 56-year-old shop assistant who consulted me with a long history of left-sided headaches with associated flashing lights and vomiting. She knew she suffered from migraine but had been unable to identify the cause. Her job was interesting with no stress involved, and her home life was happy and trouble-free. Strangely, her headaches usually started in the mornings and she never experienced them on a Sunday. This alerted me to the possibility that there was a link with the food she was eating, especially as she did not eat breakfast on Sundays. It has been shown that about 25 per cent of migraine attacks are caused by chemicals in food and these are commonly found in cheese, chocolate, fruit, coffee, and red wine. Grace didn't eat any of these for breakfast but I have also seen migraine produced by products containing wheat and corn. On eliminating breakfast cereal she stopped having the headaches.

In these three cases we have covered the main triggers of migraine in stress, drugs, and food. However, as indicated at the beginning of the chapter, it is a very individual problem and some people may have other circumstances that promote an attack. Sleeping too heavily, having a lie-in, or even any alcoholic drink are factors which can trigger migraine in an unfortunate few.

Migraine is a most miserable condition but it can be relieved or, at worst, greatly improved by simple practical steps as outlined in the section on treatment. If you are a migraine sufferer, you owe it to yourself to try it.

Sinusitis

If you suffer from frequent colds, or live in an area where the level of air pollution is high, then headaches from congestion of the sinuses are an all too common occurrence. Fumes from industry, car exhausts, cigarette smoke, dust, and pollen all combine to contaminate the atmosphere, producing the aching frontal pain of sinusitis. The sinuses are hollow, air-filled spaces in the cheekbones and the bones of the forehead, and the characteristic throbbing headaches are felt above or behind the eyes. These cavities are directly connected to the nose via narrow channels and their main function is to produce the mucus for the nasal passages. This fluid serves as a protection to the lungs by trapping any foreign particles that are breathed in. If the sinuses are irritated, either from these pollutants or from the common cold, they then secrete a vast quantity of this fluid. This excess mucus attempts to flow down the narrow channels to the nose but often these are already constricted or even blocked for the same reason that the sinus cavities are aggravated. Stagnation of the mucus results leading to infection and to back pressure in the sinus cavities. As these are surrounded by bone, they are unable to expand to ease this pressure and become very painful, producing the typical headaches.

Carol G. was a 26-year-old office worker who had experienced several colds each winter since she was a child. Each time, she went on to develop a severe throbbing ache in her forehead with a feeling of total nasal blockage. On this occasion the pain had also started in the cheekbone, and she felt thoroughly miserable. Carol had come to the surgery as her symptoms were spreading and she found this very worrying. There are several sinuses in the area of the face and forehead and you can see from the diagram that the infection had reached both her frontal and maxillary sinuses. The reason for the difference in her condition this time was that previously only the frontal sinus had been affected. Interestingly, Carol remarked that some of her teeth were aching and this arises because some of the roots of larger back teeth extend into the maxillary sinus. In fact, sinusitis sufferers sometimes make their first visit for help to their dentist rather than the doctor.

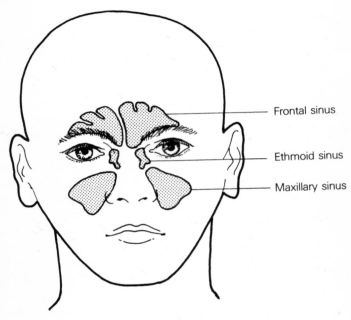

Frontal sinus

Ethmoid sinus

Maxillary sinus

Sinuses in face

On her previous visits to other doctors Carol had usually been prescribed antibiotics and decongestants without success. These, theoretically, should be effective but in practice often make the problems worse as both tend to thicken the mucus which further prevents its flow to the nose. In addition there are the inevitable side-effects as antibiotics damage the friendly bacteria in the bowel, and decongestants make you feel depressed, tired, and completely dried up. I know that the one time I took a decongestant myself I could not wait for the effect to wear off as it made me feel worse than the original condition!

The treatment of Carol's problem needed not only to be focused on immediate relief of her headaches but also on the reasons for her catching so many colds. As sinusitis develops from blockage of the channels to the nose, the logical treatment is to remove this blockage. This can be done in a rather barbaric way in hospital but I have found simple intra-nasal douches carried out regularly at home to be more effective and much less traumatic. More information on wash-outs is given in Chapter 8. When Carol was shown the technique her headaches quickly disappeared. Furthermore, she developed greater confidence for future attacks as she now knew there was an effective method of alleviating them.

Her low resistance to simple infections was caused by a suppression of her immune system during the winter months. Since Carol was very sensitive to cold weather, as a protective reflex her diet contained more fat and she tended to eat snacks between meals. In summer, regular tennis maintained her fitness but in winter the courts were closed and exercise became virtually nonexistent. This combination of poor diet and no physical exertion was sufficient to lower her immune system. Simple correction of these problems was all that was needed in this case.

Carol's problem was a classical sinus headache which she was able to relieve by straightforward steps at home and which did not involve the use of drugs. Of course not everyone is so fortunate, and management can be more complex, as in James T.'s situation below.

James T. was a 48-year-old financier who worked in a busy stockbrokers' office. His was a high pressure job which he enjoyed and to counter this pressure he ate a healthy low-fat diet and took regular exercise. His main problem was the extremely smoky atmosphere at work, which produced a persistent frontal headache after a couple of hours. Although he was a non-smoker, the passively inhaled fumes had caused his sinus passages to swell, creating back pressure and the resultant headaches. James's requests for a clearer atmosphere had fallen on deaf ears, as his colleagues found that cigarettes eased the tension of the job. The main difficulty, therefore, was that the direct cause of the sinus headaches could not be removed or even lessened. He was averse to taking painkillers and had found that decongestants destroyed his concentration at a time when he needed to be at his most alert.

The aim of treatment in this situation is to widen out the sinus channels, thus counteracting the effect of the smoke. This must be done without producing any side-effects, and alternative medical techniques are ideal. I started James on a short course of acupuncture and then taught him a technique called acupressure which is easy to learn and enabled him to treat himself whenever the headache occurred. Combined with homoeopathic tablets this regime proved most effective and his headaches subsided.

This case history is important because whilst it is always ideal to eliminate the underlying cause, this is not always possible. Please do not despair if you fall into this category, as by using relatively simple methods the headaches can be completely eradicated. These methods are explained in detail in the section on treatment.

High blood pressure

Headaches can be an early warning sign of raised blood pressure. The heart's main function is to pump the blood around the body along a network of blood vessels. These arteries and veins are like a series of pipes and if they narrow for any reason the heart has to work at an increased pressure to force the same amount of blood down them. If the heart has to beat at high pressure for any length of time it will weaken and eventually fail, leading to premature death. The cause of an increase in blood pressure is a mystery, but research shows that once blood pressure is returned to a normal level, life expectancy is not reduced.

The problem with high blood pressure is that it can be of insidious onset with few symptoms, and nowadays everyone is urged to have a yearly check at their doctor's surgery. The first manifestation is usually a severe throbbing headache situated at the back of the head. It is unusual in that it is worse on waking whereas headaches from other causes are relieved by sleep. Dizziness, weakness, blurred vision and palpitations are other features, but it is interesting that the majority of these occur *after* the diagnosis of high blood pressure has been made!

Brenda G. was a 51-year-old woman who had her own business running a local day nursery. She was highly successful and had a long waiting list of children for entry. There was a considerable amount of stress with the job, and she had always suffered with classical tension headaches. More recently, however, their nature had changed as they were more painful and had moved to the back of the head. Whereas her tension headaches had always worsened throughout the day, these were present immediately on waking. Brenda commented that at times her head felt like a pressure cooker which was about to explode. Physical examination was normal except that her blood pressure was markedly raised. Sometimes this may only be temporary so it is always necessary to recheck it on several occasions to ensure that the high level is constant. Unfortunately for Brenda, her reading was consistently above the top limit and it would not have been safe to ignore it.

It is not known why some people have a tendency for their blood pressure to rise, but there are certain lifestyle factors that influence it. Brenda had a stressful occupation, liked a cigarette or two at the end of the day and was carrying a stone in extra weight. She admitted to adding salt to her food at mealtimes and always put some in her cooking. Stress, smoking, obesity and salt are all well-recognized risk factors and it was important that Brenda corrected these before drug therapy was considered. As the adverse effects of high blood pressure are slow to develop, treatment must not be rushed into too quickly as, once started, drugs need to be taken for life. Happily, by improving her lifestyle Brenda reduced her blood pressure to below the level requiring treatment and now she just calls in at the surgery every few months for a routine check.

Blood pressure does tend to increase with age and sometimes this can present problems. Joan B. was a 57-year-old machinist in the local silk factory who had been discovered to have raised blood pressure fifteen years previously. She had eliminated all her risk factors and had done extremely well to avoid medication all that time. In the last few weeks Joan had developed persistent headaches which she could not localize to any particular area. She was dizzy at times and felt nauseous. I had warned her that these were symptoms that would indicate that her blood pressure was increasing. Measurement confirmed that the level was creeping up and that further measures needed to be taken to lower it. I could tell by the fearful look in Joan's eyes that she expected me to start her on drugs.

Fortunately, high blood pressure is one of the few situations in medicine where it is not imperative to reverse the condition rapidly. The harmful effects only develop slowly over a number of years, and therefore it is wrong to overreact and introduce therapy that may be too strong and even unnecessary. I am not saying that there is never a case for using drugs, but I feel strongly that all other methods should be tried first. Every drug has some side-effects and those for controlling blood pressure are no exception. These include tiredness, weakness of limbs, dizziness from lowering the blood pressure too much, reduction of sex drive, and impotence in men. These ill-effects are uncommon and I would not wish to worry anyone already on drugs, but it just wouldn't appeal to me to have to start on something I would have to take for the rest of my life.

Joan was also very much against commencing drug treatment, and was delighted that there were other possibilities. Her headaches, although a nuisance, were at a tolerable level and did not require painkillers. Whilst she did not lead a particularly stressful life, it has been shown that practising relaxation methods regularly has a marked effect on lowering blood pressure. This involves setting aside about 20 minutes every day for this purpose in a quiet and peaceful location. I lent Joan a relaxation cassette and she soon mastered the technique. An extension of this, which I will enlarge on in Chapters 8 and 11, is to learn self-hypnosis. The hypnotic state is a changed level of consciousness somewhere between being awake and being asleep. It is simple to learn, and very deep levels of relaxation can be achieved.

Another important self-help approach to use is special breathing exercises. These help to expand the lungs more fully and thus increase the uptake of oxygen into the blood. This means the heart does not have to pump as much blood around the body, and the blood pressure therefore falls. Again these are easy exercises to learn and can be combined quite easily with the relaxation.

Joan did extremely well at both relaxation and breathing. She did however need to combine these with regular exercise and in particular walking. This is a steady gradual physical activity which is particularly beneficial to the heart muscles. The improved efficiency of these muscles means they do not have to work as hard and there is a consequence drop in blood pressure.

I stressed again the importance of a low-fat diet to Joan, as fats can damage the blood vessel walls, and told her that she had to limit her intake of alcohol. There are an array of supplements that can be taken, including different vitamins and chemicals. In Joan's situation I recommended eight brewer's yeast tablets a day and two garlic capsules.

Happily, her blood pressure came down to normal, although it had taken considerable effort and discipline on Joan's part. However, it had been well worth it as she had avoided any drug therapy. With the fall in pressure her headaches completely disappeared and hopefully will never return. Should there ever be any further problems, the next course of action would be homoeopathic tablets which can be very successful.

Headaches are a cardinal sign of high blood pressure and this is another reason why they should not merely be suppressed with painkillers. It is always vital to ascertain the cause of a continual headache as only then can the appropriate remedial action be taken. As illustrated by the cases above, even if it is a symptom of a potentially serious condition it can still be treated by simple and natural methods. I will deal with the treatment in detail later in the book.

Other causes

While tension, migraine, sinusitis and high blood pressure represent the vast majority of headaches, this will be of no consolation to you if your own headaches do not fall into one of these categories. The object of this section is to illustrate the other causes which, although not as common, are just as significant and equally disabling. By the end of this chapter everyone should be in a position to identify the reason for their own particular headache. This is vital as it makes management easier and more precise.

Cervical spondylitis

Gladys R. was a 69-year-old retired woman whom I had seen at the surgery for several years with arthritis of the hips. On one of her visits she complained of headaches associated with dizziness. She told me these started at the back of the neck and spread over her scalp to the forehead. The pain was quite sharp and became worse when she moved her head and in particular when she turned to one side. She had also noticed some tingling in her arms and hands which was quite distressing. The headaches could last for several hours and were not relieved by simple painkillers. Gladys' description fitted the type of headache which is referred from the bones in her neck which had plainly, like her hips, become affected by arthritis. This is known medically as cervical spondylitis. Arthritis is really wear and tear of the bones as you become older and this produces irritation and swelling around the affected joints. It is this swelling that usually produces the pain and, by pressing on various nerves, causes pins and needles and the characteristic crippling headaches.

Gladys was most concerned at this new development, but I was able to reassure her that cervical spondylitis does not become too disabling as long as the correct approach is taken. While there is no specific cure for arthritis, the aim of therapy is to reduce the swelling around the affected part. This then relieves the pressure on the nerves, and the pain and headaches will disappear. For Gladys I prescribed a cervical collar to immobilize her neck and thus allow the joints to rest. This is of most value at night, when involuntary movements tend to occur — anyway she was not keen to wear one in the daytime. A course of therapy from an osteopath or chiropractor is the most effective treatment and, in four weeks, Gladys' headaches had completely disappeared. Physiotherapy or acupuncture would have been reasonable alternatives, but I have always found the others to be quicker and longer-lasting.

Eye problems

In the surgery I am increasingly finding that persistent headaches are related to the eyes. Sarah H. was a 17-year-old college student who suffered from pain in the forehead which invariably started about 3 o'clock in the afternoon. It never developed at weekends and her mother wondered if the pressure of work was proving too much for Sarah. The site of the headaches did not support this theory, so I wondered if a problem with the eyes was the cause. Although she denied any visual symptoms, simple testing showed her to be very short-sighted. This meant that the muscles of the eyes were having to work much harder to focus. Towards the end of the day these muscles became fatigued and the headache resulted. Both the headaches and her schoolwork improved dramatically with the appropriate glasses.

Headache from eye-strain is common in teenagers and young adults but in older people it is usually from glaucoma. Doris R. was a 76-year-old woman who developed severe pain behind the left eye which seemed to go right through her head. Her eyes were extremely sensitive to light. Now, the inner part of the eye is bathed in a watery fluid and this drains away down narrow channels. Sometimes as age progresses these become blocked and the pressure of fluid builds up. This causes pain and head-aches and ultimately, if untreated can lead to blindness. On gently palpating Doris' eye I discovered that the pressure was very high, but I was able to start her on some eye drops which quickly relieved it, leading to the disappearance of her headaches. Not all cases of glaucoma are so obvious but all opticians have machines for measuring eye pressure so it is easy to diagnose.

Infections

Any infection which cases a rise in temperature can produce generalized headaches. Wayne Y., aged 7, was seen on a home visit with a temperature of 104 degrees and a cough which he had had for three days. I asked his parents why they had not brought him to the surgery and they said they were worried about menin-gitis, as he was crying with pains in his head. On examining him I found that Wayne had an acute tonsillitis, which was sufficient to cause his pyrexia (fever), cough and headache. Meningitis could be ruled out as this produces marked neck stiffness so the head cannot be raised off the pillow or turned to the side. Also, the headache is usually confined to the back of the head and neck. I am happy to say that Wayne recovered without treatment in a few days.

Teeth

Not being a dental expert, I puzzled for some time last year over Deborah H. who had persistent frontal headaches. They did not really fit the pattern of either migraine or sinusitis but she did comment that over the years she had experienced considerable trouble with her teeth. It seemed to me that her bite was abnormal and that this was throwing extra strain on the joint between the jaw and the skull. I referred her to her dentist who corrected this problem and her headaches were relieved. Even though nobody likes going, it is always worth a trip to the dentist for an unexplained headache or facial pain.

Trauma

This may sound an incredibly obvious cause of headaches, but it is amazing the number of people I see in the surgery who never think to mention that they have received a blow to the head. Headaches caused by trauma can persist for weeks or months and are often produced by a relatively minor injury. More serious trauma can cause concussion, which is basically a 'shaking up' of the brain, and this also can result in a generalized headache lasting intermittently for several months.

Rarer, more serious causes

I have deliberately left this group to the last as they are so uncommon that I did not want undue emphasis placed on them. I suppose many people fear a brain tumour but in eleven years in general practice I have only seen one. Contrast that with the three cases of headache I see every surgery, and I hope it puts it into perspective.

The presenting features of a brain tumour usually follow the classical pattern. Susan A. was a 38-year-old woman who had complained of headaches for three months. She could not local-ize them and they had increased in severity until they almost made her scream. Coupled with that, she had started to vomit and had developed marked sensitivity to light. Her vision had become blurred, and examining her eyes showed a marked increase in pressure. This triad of symptoms consisting of generalized head-ache, vomiting and sensitivity to light is typical of raised intra-cranial pressure usually caused by a tumour. However, that does not necessarily mean the beginning of the end, as many tumours are now treatable. Happily, Susan's turned out to be a non-cancerous growth and was removed, following which she made a full recovery.

The bursting of a blood vessel within the brain is another unusual presentation of headaches. Tony M. was a 45-year-old builder who was out shopping when he felt as though he had been suddenly punched on the back of the neck. He staggered, but did not fall down, and recovered enough to return home. Over the next few hours his headache became localized to the back of the head and he developed severe neck stiffness. He became confused and, although conscious, was not aware of his surroundings. Tony had suffered a sub-arachnoid haemorrhage, which is where an artery bursts in a particular part of the brain. This is a life-threatening condition and I admitted Tony to hospital immediately. After preliminary tests an operation was performed to tie off the offending vessel and he made an uneventful return to normal health.

There is one other important disease that may cause headaches and that is called temporal (cranial) arteritis. Celia T. was 61 years of age and went to her doctor with increasing headache over her right temple and sudden deterioration in vision. On examination she was extremely tender over one of the blood vessels of the temple and this vessel felt thickened and inflamed. The cause of this condition is unknown but it is important because if ignored it can spread to the arteries in the eye producing sudden blindness. However, once I started Celia on some treatment the risk of that disappeared and she quickly recovered.

Please do not be too concerned that you might have one of the three conditions above as I stress again that they are all extremely rare. However, if you are worried, then your doctor will easily be able to test for these and thus reassure you.

Summary charts

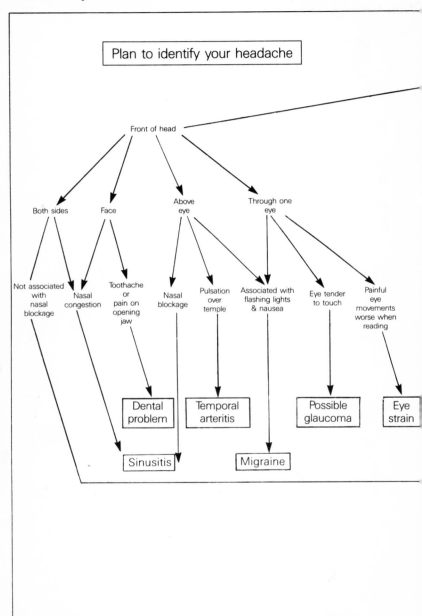

Plan to identify your headache

Front of head

Both sides • Face • Above eye • Through one eye

Not associated with nasal blockage • Nasal congestion • Toothache or pain on opening jaw • Nasal blockage • Pulsation over temple • Associated with flashing lights & nausea • Eye tender to touch • Painful eye movements worse when reading

Dental problem • Temporal arteritis • Possible glaucoma • Eye strain

Sinusitis • Migraine

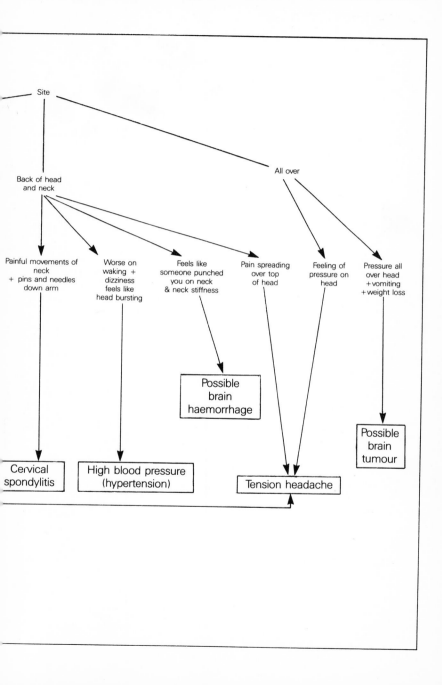

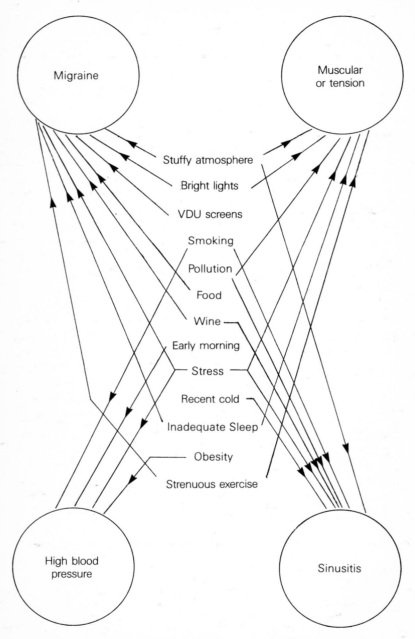

Precipitating factors in the major causes of headaches

CHAPTER 2

The immune system

Twenty-four hours a day, every day of our lives, there is a defence mechanism within the body ready to fight off harmful situations. This is called the immune system, and most people take it for granted as part of our natural bodily processes. However, nowadays more than ever, the immune system is under continual pressure from an increasing array of infections and numerous environmental influences. Unless steps are taken to keep the system in tip-top condition, the pressure on it may become too great and its efficiency thereby will be severely compromised. Once this occurs it cannot be relied upon and the individual becomes open to headaches, recurrent flu, colds, chronic fatigue and even more serious health problems like cancer.

Maintaining an excellent immune system is the whole crux of medicine and this is why health magazines are always stressing ways to improve it. Unfortunately they never describe its composition, or how it actually works, and patients often ask me to explain the system to them. A typical example was the case of Kate B., a 34-year-old woman who came to the surgery with persistent and very troublesome tension headaches. The feeling of a heavy weight pressing down on her head was relentless and had been slowly worsening over several months. During the same period of time she had developed three episodes of tonsillitis, an infection in her urine and her skin had become spotty. To add to the situation her periods had become irregular and her premenstrual tension more pronounced. The headaches before her periods were unbearable and almost made her scream. Kate had a daughter aged 2 and a year before, in partnership with a friend, had opened a day nursery. This had proved much harder work than anticipated, as anyone who has started a new business will realize. It had seemed a good idea originally, as she could keep her own child with her at the nursery, but recently Kate had started to worry that her daughter was becoming institution-alized. To further increase the tension, her husband, an insurance broker, had been made redundant and had decided to start up on his own.

Stress

I explained to Kate that her health problems were the result of all the stress she had been through with looking after a small child, starting a new business and the financial trauma of her husband's loss of income. The position was not helped either by her continual exposure to minor infections from the other children at the nursery. Both stress and infection will drain the immune system and leave the individual much more open to conditions like headaches. Kate looked a little disbelieving and commented that whilst she had heard of the immune system, that was as far as her knowledge went. I therefore set out to explain it and to convince her that its suppression was the root cause of her ill-health.

The immune system is in many ways like a rail network, consisting of a series of tubes which supply every part of the body in the same way that railway lines serve each area of the country. At various points along the route there are stopping points. On the railway, these are stations, but in the body they are called lymph glands and each group of glands serves its own particular section. I am sure everyone knows that when you develop a throat infection or catch a cold the glands in the neck swell up. There are similar groups of glands all over the body and they all react if challenged by infection or trauma. If for example, a toe becomes infected it will lead to enlarged glands in the groin; similarly, a cut on the hand brings up glands in the armpit. Once they have swollen, it takes several weeks for them to return to normal size, often long after the infection has disappeared. Kate confirmed that the glands under her chin were nearly always enlarged and painful, and I explained that this was because they had insufficient time to recover between infections.

Lymphocytes

The body can be invaded by a wide range of foreign matter. This may be from viruses and bacteria, cancer cells, incompatible blood transfusions, transplants, or even small pieces of grit in a cut. When this assault occurs, there are certain cells in the body which will fight and destroy the attackers. These are called white blood cells, of which there are several different kinds: the most important are known as *lymphocytes*. They are produced by the bone marrow, which is in the centre of the major bones of the body, and also by the spleen.

I tried to clarify the actual steps that occur with special reference to Kate's own throat. When the infection is caught, lymphocytes that have been produced by the bone marrow and spleen pass in the bloodstream to the tonsils where they set about the invading viruses. Once the viruses have been killed or neutralized they are taken into the 'rail system', in this case the lymph channels, and transported to the lymph glands in the neck where they are completely broken down.

Kate was happy with this explanation although she realized it was an oversimplification and as it was the end of that particular consultation I arranged to see her again in a week. However, her inquisitive mind took her to the local library the following day to read further on the subject. At her next appointment she was a little worried as she had discovered that a deficiency of certain types of lymphocytes can actually cause cancer. In fact, this is a distortion of the truth, but naturally the fear of developing cancer had increased her stress, thereby worsening her headaches. Kate asked me to explain it in more detail so she would not be worried.

As mentioned above, the main constituent of the defence system is the lymphocyte, of which there are two types: the B lymphocyte and the T lymphocyte. These are present both in the blood and in lymph nodes. These cells are highly mobile and will move quickly around the body to wherever they are required and in Kate's situation to her throat. There are always a certain number of each type of lymphocyte in the body, and they are capable of extremely fast reproduction when they come into contact with foreign material. At any one time there can be millions of them fighting the attackers. Although these lymphocytes all appear the same, they have an amazing number of minor variations which ensure that there are always certain ones that are suited to any particular invader. In tonsil infections it is usually the lymphocytes that act against viruses that are required.

Kate had read in the library that it was her T lymphocytes that were deficient and she wondered why one type was different from the other. In fact they work in different ways, although their actions are closely linked. The B lymphocytes are effective by producing substances called antibodies which are of infinite variety, each one being able to deal with one particular kind of foreign invader.

Let us consider a case of measles. When this develops, it takes the body a few days to produce the appropriate antibodies, so the initial infection is quite severe. The antibodies, when formed, then destroy the viruses and the child recovers. A few of the antibodies will always remain in the body so if, later in life, the person is exposed to the measles virus again, then these antibodies rapidly multiply and destroy the virus, preventing reinfection.

Unfortunately, some foreign invaders are too strong or unsuitable for the antibodies to kill, and this is where the T lymphocytes come into their own. They work by directly attacking the invading cells, adhering to their surface and destroying them. It takes large numbers to do this and the body is able under normal circumstances to produce T lymphocytes at a rate of 2,000 per second.

I stressed to Kate that this healing process using lymphocytes is incredibly effective, and far more complex than anything science could ever invent. So why is it then that we still catch infections and suffer from serious diseases like cancer? The simple reason is that illness develops because the immune system is not able to work at full efficiency. This loss of power is not present at birth and must therefore be acquired at some point.

The thymus gland

In the front of the neck there is a small organ called the thymus gland, which is of great importance as it is the place in which the lymphocytes acquire their individuality and where they multiply and mature. Without a thymus, although there would be lymphocytes in the body, they would not be specific enough or in sufficient quantity to prevent disease from developing. The thymus reaches maximum size soon after puberty and then over the years it slowly shrinks until, in old age, it may be difficult to locate. It is logical, therefore, that as age progresses everyone's natural resistance to illness weakens, but this is only part of the story. It has been shown that there are many controllable factors which encourage shrinkage of the thymus gland and consequently a lowering of immunity.

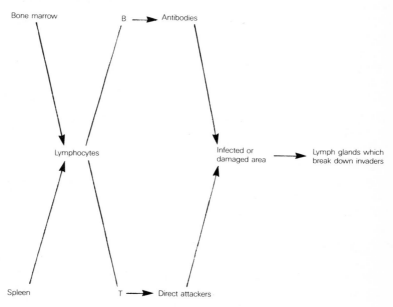

Mechanism of the immune system

First in line are the dreaded side-effects of some drugs and, in particular, the use of steroids or cortisone. Whilst I appreciate that cortisone can be a life-saver, it should never be used except in severe conditions because of its effect on the thymus. This drug is by no means the only one associated with immune deficiency and even prolonged used of antibiotics can impair immunity.

In the past ten years it has become more and more evident that it is often quite simple circumstances which suppress the immune system. Pollution and our noisy crowded environment can all take their toll. So can the things we do to ourselves, such as smoking, eating the wrong foods, and denying ourselves the sleep, relaxation and exercise our bodies need. Our state of mind also plays a large part. It is no coincidence that annoying problems like headaches, thrush, rashes, boils and stomach problems crop up when we are feeling low. When we are depressed or not taking care of ourselves our immune system is laid low too, leaving us wide open to all kinds of illness and infection.

Ways of boosting your immune system
1) Wholefood diet
2) Regular exercise
3) Control of stress

Ways of depressing your immune system
1) Drugs
2) Pollution
3) Smoking
4) Inadequate sleep
5) Poor diet
6) Lack of exercise
7) High stress level and inadequate relaxation

By far the most important of the factors suppressing the immune system, however, is stress. Everyone suffers from stress to differing degrees; and unless ways are actively undertaken to control it, it can wreak havoc on the immune system. Recent research at Cambridge showed that the herpes virus responsible for cold sores is more active in students under stress because of examinations. Five years ago many people felt that admitting to stress was a sign of weakness, but fortunately that attitude is rapidly changing.

Kate was still concerned about the link with cancer and it is certainly true that in certain types of cancer there has been shown to be a marked reduction in T lymphocytes. These lymphocytes would normally destroy the cancer cells, but obviously if there are not many of them about, then the malignant cells may develop a hold. It is significant also that people can often date the development of this condition to a particularly stressful experience like a bereavement or divorce.

Kate looked horrified, but I was quickly able to reassure her that it works the other way round as well, in that she can boost her own immune system and help it to fight off illness and infection. In her own case the lifestyle she was leading, being very stressful, was suppressing the production of her lymphocytes and allowing throat infections and her constant headaches to persist. Over the following chapters I have outlined the steps that must be taken to stimulate and then maintain the immune system in perfect condition. I firmly believe that the chance of contracting a serious illness is then virtually negligible. Happily, Kate has adhered to these principles and her headaches and sore throats have completely disappeared.

Boosting your immune system

CHAPTER 3

Eating the right food

Wouldn't it be fantastic if we could eat anything we felt like without having to worry about the effect on our bodies? Indeed, this attitude has prevailed in Britain for many years, so it is not surprising that the British are near the top of the league for ill-health in the civilized world. All nations that have produced a programme for healthy eating have noticed a sharp fall not only in the serious conditions like heart disease but also in the numerous minor ailments. The quality of our life depends on keeping well, and this in itself is largely determined by the quality of food we eat. It can make the difference between feeling lively and energetic all day or being so exhausted at the end of work that you fall asleep in the chair on arrival home. The main effect of a poor quality diet is that it suppresses the immune system, making it difficult to eradicate the minor illnesses that a flourishing system would normally destroy very quickly.

Headache is one of the first symptoms of an immune system in poor condition, and therefore it is vital that headache sufferers do everything possible to boost their immune system. A balanced and healthy diet will play a major role in achieving this. Unfortunately, it is not always easy to accomplish, as there is an ever-growing list of so-called foods marketed solely to make money. The manufacturers of these products have not the slightest interest in their depressant effect on the immune system and the resultant illnesses they produce in children and adults. Indeed, most of these manufactuers deny that food and illness have any connection, even though scientific evidence is overwhelming. If good health is to be achieved then poor quality food must be avoided and the level of immune-strengthening nutrients must be high.

Often the objection to a healthy diet is that it is expensive, but in fact the reverse is true. Money is not wasted on junk food and naturally there are no dental bills! The problem is that many people do squander their money on foods which can never produce good health. At least two-thirds of the food in the supermarkets is not worth carrying home, let alone paying for!

There is a bewildering amount of information written on diet and it is often difficult to understand or so complicated that it is impossible to apply in practice. By reading this chapter you will have a good basic knowledge of the constitution of food and of the simple steps you can take to achieve a healthy balance in your eating habits.

A healthy balance

Barry L. was a 37-year-old taxi driver who had recently developed irritating tension headaches which were affecting his driving. His lifestyle was deficient in that he took little exercise and was four stone overweight. I started to explain to him that his headaches were a result of these factors and that his food intake was too high in fats and too low in protein. However, when I pointed this out to him he shrugged his shoulders and said he had no idea what the difference was between them. My sympathy was certainly with him as I remember when I was a medical student being on a ward round with a very intimidating consultant. We were discussing a patient with malnutrition and suddenly he turned to me and asked me the difference in function between carbohydrate, fats and protein. With a bright red face I was forced to admit that I had no real idea, and he sent me off the ward to visit the hospital dietitian for a lesson. I could hear all the nurses laughing in the background!

Food, I told Barry, is made up of four basic nutrients. **Carbohydrate,** which is the chief source of energy but in excess can be converted to fat; **protein,** which is responsible for growth and repair of the body; **fat,** which has an insulating and protective function but in excess makes you overweight; and **vitamins,** which are responsible for the life and well-being of the body. If these are maintained at optimum levels then good health will automatically follow, but I explained to Barry that his nutrient levels had become unbalanced and this was the reason for his headaches. Unfortunately, much of his diet was convenience food out of tins and these contain other substances such as colourants, flavourings and preservatives. These fulfil merely a promotional function in making the food seem more interesting, and in excess can damage the immune system making the headaches worse. Barry was obviously very interested so I went into more detail.

Carbohydrate

Carbohydrate provides most of the energy needed by the body and in Britain more carbohydrate than either fat or protein is consumed. Everything living requires energy to function and if insufficient is obtained from the diet then the body will slow down and become lethargic. Should this continue, as it often does in Third World countries, then death will eventually result. All carbohydrates originate from plants as these contain chlorophyll which can absorb energy from the sun. Most of this energy is stored and is available to us as food if we eat cereals like wheat, tubers (usually as potatoes), and root crops such as sugar beet.

When these carbohydrates are eaten they pass through the stomach into the intestine where they are all converted to sugar. There are several types of sugar but the important one to remember is glucose, as it is this that the body uses to provide energy. They are then absorbed into the bloodstream where the insulin determines how much glucose stays in the blood and how much is stored as fat. (In people with diabetes, there is a deficiency of insulin and too much sugar builds up in the blood.) I explained to Barry that in his diet he was taking in too much sugar for his energy requirements and this was being converted to fat.

Protein

Protein has a different role from carbohydrate as it provides the means for growth and repair. The body is made up of millions and millions of cells joined together, and only protein can form new ones. Thus our muscles, bones, skin, hair and internal organs all require adequate supplies of protein to maintain themselves, and this can only be obtained from food. Obviously, it is important for children to have an adequate supply, as they are continually growing, but it is equally vital for adults, as parts of the body are constantly wearing out and need replenishing. Amazingly, a structure like the heart needs complete replacement of its cells about every 20 days.

When protein is eaten, it is broken down in the intestine into structures called amino acids. These are absorbed into the blood where they are regrouped to form the various types of protein required to build each individual kind of body tissue. As these amino acids cannot be stored in the body for any length of time, it is necessary that an assortment is provided at each meal so that they are all available.

Barry commented at this point that the reason he didn't eat enough protein was because he was unable to afford red meat. I am sure he was thinking of the weightlifters you see on the television who eat six steaks a day! I was able to assure him that, similarly to carbohydrate, all protein starts initially in plants and it is therefore quite possible to take an adequate amount in the diet from vegetarian sources.

Fats

The mention of the word *fats* definitely made Barry feel uneasy as he was carrying far too much! The main function of fat is as a store of energy and any surplus food we eat, of whatever nature, is converted into fat and stored as a layer mainly under the skin. This can then be used for energy if required. If you are on a diet to lose weight the aim is to take in less energy in the food than is needed for everyday living. The body then has to break down its own fat to obtain this energy and over a period of time weight is lost. Many fats in food are obvious, such as fat on meat, butter and cooking oil, but others are more obscure and are called 'invisible'. These occur in eggs, nuts, milk, cakes, chocolate, pastries and in many other foods. They can be further subdivided into saturated and unsaturated fat, and it is the former kind that is linked with heart disease. Most people eat far too much fat, which is usually of the saturated type, but a small amount of unsaturated fat is actually beneficial as it keeps down the level of cholesterol, thus preventing heart disease. Further functions are in binding the body cells together, supporting various structures such as the kidneys which actually sit in a pillow of fat, and also forming an insulating layer beneath the skin against cold temperatures.

Barry was a little irritated by my comments on his weight, so although he accepted my explanation of his nutrition, he said he could not see that it had any relation to his headaches, which was the reason he had come to see me in the first place. I stressed to him that his headaches were caused by the poor condition of his immune system. This system requires adequate carbohydrate to give it energy to fight off illness, sufficient protein to allow it to keep itself in excellent repair, and enough unsaturated fat to support its cell structure and to give it a reserve energy supply.

Vitamins

He could see the logic of this and readily admitted that his own diet was both unbalanced and inadequate. This led on to the fourth constituent of food which are the *vitamins*. These are a group of substances which are essential for the life and well-being of our body. We only need minute amounts, but, with the present methods of preserving food, these vitamins can often be lost. There are a tremendous number of vitamins and obviously it is impossible to take supplements of all of them. As we are concerned in this book with curing headaches by boosting the immune system I will only mention the three vitamins which have been shown to do this:

Vitamin A is found in milk, eggs, and red vegetables such as carrots. This vitamin keeps the skin healthy, which is necessary as it is the first line of defence in the body's immune system, repelling invaders before they have the opportunity to take hold.

The **B vitamins** are a group of vitamins found in wholegrain cereals, yeast and green leafy vegetables. Deficiency in these vitamins reduces the immune antibody response, making the body less able to react quickly to invading infections.

Thirdly, **vitamin C,** found in fresh fruit and vegetables, is one of the vital vitamins for the immune system as it helps the body to fight off bacteria and viruses. In addition it increases the ability to capture and destroy any infections that actually gain a hold on the body. I would certainly recommend to everyone that they take sufficient of each of these vitamins in their food every day.

A little further on in this chapter you will find the necessary steps to take to achieve a balanced and healthy diet, and I am happy to say that Barry followed these most diligently. He looks and feels much healthier and his headaches have disappeared.

Maureen L. was a 31-year-old woman who came to see me with a history of persistent headaches which usually started in the

neck and swept over the top of the scalp to the forehead. Sometimes they were one-sided and associated with nausea and vomiting and just occasionally they were in the face associated with
nasal congestion. This was an apparently confusing picture, and
in fact she was suffering from three different kinds of headaches:
muscular, migraine and sinusitis. I suspected that her immune
system was not functioning normally, and questioned her on her
lifestyle. Maureen worked as a waitress in a local fast food restaur-
ant, which involved long, irregular hours, and at the end of her
shift she was able to have a free meal. Hamburgers, chips and a
fizzy drink were the normal fare and this rarely varied. Maureen
knew that this was not a healthy diet, and was quite relieved when
I explained this was the reason for her headaches. She had been
convinced that a brain tumour was the underlying cause and her
life was in danger. Most people have no real idea how to change
to healthy food, or indeed what it consists of, and Maureen was
no exception. She understood already about protein, fat and
carbohydrate but found talk of 'wholefoods' rather confusing.

Wholefoods

Everyone should be on a wholefood diet, and there is no need to
be worried or put off by the name. It simply means foods that have
nothing added to them and nothing taken away. They are not pro-
cessed or refined and are near as possible to their natural state. No
additives like flavourings, colourings or preservatives can have
been added as these have a direct depressant effect on the immune
system. Wholefoods are important as they contain the nutrients
we need, in a form we can use. An example of this is wholemeal
bread which is made from unrefined flour and contains natural
wheat bran which is a type of fibre. It is also packed with B vitamins and several minerals. To make white bread the flour is
refined, and in this process it loses most of its vitamins, minerals and fibre. Fibre is important as a filler thus preventing us
from overeating, helping digestion, and regulating the bowels.
Maureen had noticed how easy it is to eat slice after slice of
fibreless white bread compared with nourishing, filling wholemeal bread. A diet of refined foods results in people who are
overfed and undernourished, and who lack the vitamins necessary for vitality.

Eating foods as near to their natural state as possible has a number of beneficial effects on the immune system. Processing and cooking destroy many of the nutrients in food which are essential for good health. Additives are only needed because we've come to expect the extra taste, and as a general rule I feel that if the food needs disguising to make it palatable, then it is better not eaten at all. This particularly applies to convenience foods like beefburgers which are usually made from different parts of the body as diverse as brain and spleen. This creates a bizarre taste, and to make them palatable and pleasing to look at they are packed full of flavourings and colourants. Maureen was turning a strange shade of green at the thought of her daily helping but at least it seemed to be shocking her into action! In fact, quite apart from all the additives she was eating, a diet containing too much meat can be harmful as it contains a considerable amount of saturated fat. Vegetarians statistically suffer from fewer heart attacks than meat eaters. It is not essential on a wholefood diet to cut out meat completely, but restrict it to twice a week and choose the leanest cuts or white meat like chicken.

All food starts in the ground, whether it is eaten directly by us or consumed by animals first, so if the soil is deficient then so is the food we eat. Underfed crops don't grow properly and are then prone to disease and pests. To counteract this problem, farmers add excessive fertilizers to the soil and spray the crops with pesticides. Both of these can be left on the food in sufficient quantity to cause a harmful effect on the immune system when eaten. In view of this it is wise to eat organically grown crops to which nothing has been added. Unfortunately, many farms are jumping on the bandwagon and advertising organically grown food when in reality it takes up to ten years for all the harmful chemicals to disappear from the soil.

In brief, then, a healthy diet is one with a balance in carbohydrate and protein which is low in fat. It should consist of wholefood, i.e. food that is unrefined with no additives. Meat should be restricted, and the diet should contain plenty of fresh, organically grown vegetables and fruit. As cooking destroys vitamins and minerals, as much raw food as possible should be included. Maureen was very happy to try this as she realized that by boosting her immune system she would easily eliminate her headaches.

She asked me to write down a practical plan for her to follow and I was happy to do this.

Basic eating plan

Breakfast

Breakfast is most important as the body requires an input of energy to meet the needs for the coming day. This meal should therefore be based on starches as these are the main source of energy. However, it should not consist mainly of actual sugar because the energy from this will be used up too quickly, as illustrated in the next case. The starches should be unrefined to ensure that all the nutrients have been retained. Wholemeal bread and a wholegrain breakfast cereal like muesli will provide an excellent supply. Many cereals sold in the shops have far too much sugar added, and their energy supply is therefore too transient. Maureen was unsure if she would be able to eat muesli every day, but I suggested that natural yoghurt or fruit juice taken with it makes the muesli much more palatable. Porridge is a worthy alternative, as it contains considerable fibre which will lower the blood cholesterol. For a cooked breakfast a free-range egg — scrambled, poached or boiled — is suitable, but without added salt or butter. Fresh fruit such as grapefruit or a dried fruit compote make a superb start to the day, and either squeezed fruit juice or skimmed milk are suitable drinks.

Lunch

With sufficient energy from breakfast for most of the day, lunch is a good time to have a salad containing, where possible, a wide variety of root and leaf vegetables plus protein in the form of nuts or pulses. If you eat at work, the salad can be taken in wholemeal sandwiches and can be followed by fruit. This meal of raw, fresh food will provide a first-class supply of vitamins and minerals.

Dinner

Dinner should be based on protein, and choice can be made from lean meat, poultry, fish or a combination of the plant proteins — nuts, grains or pulses. This will then include rice dishes such as risotto or curry and wholemeal pasta such as spaghetti or maca-roni. These can be served with a raw vegetable salad or lightly steamed vegetables. For dessert I suggested fresh fruit or yoghurt or, something more substantial, a light pudding such as pancakes or mousses, made with wholemeal ingredients.

Maureen asked about drinks and I advised mineral water, fresh fruit juice, decaffeinated coffee or dry white wine but in the latter case not more than two glasses a day!

This is a basic eating plan which will set everyone on the road to good health. It is, however, a tremendous task to change the dietary habits of a lifetime, and nobody can do it without an occa-sional lapse. Never feel guilty or upset about this; if you feel like gorging yourself occasionally on cakes or chocolate, that's fine, but then go back to the job of becoming fit and healthy. The reason many people fail on different diets is that they jump in at the deep end, making a complete change to their eating habits. Some people can manage this: these are the lucky ones, but usually it is better to start slowly by changing one meal at a time. Maureen decided that breakfast would be altered first and she was happy that at last there was a practical plan she could follow. I was pleased to learn at our next consultation that her headaches had disappeared within a week of this change.

Norma H. was a 42-year-old woman who came to the surgery complaining of right-sided headaches associated with nausea, vomiting and flashing lights. These were a classical form of migraine and I proceeded to look for any precipitating factors. As migraine is often related to foodstuffs, it is important to examine the diet. Norma worked as a packer in a local chemical factory and because of family commitments she was usually on the early shift starting at 6 o'clock in the morning. Breakfast was a hurried cup of sugary coffee with a Mars bar at her first tea-break. Norma was usually too tired to make herself lunch when she came home, so her first real food of the day would be about 7 o'clock in the evening with her family. Her headaches would start about late morning and would often continue throughout the day.

I explained to Norma that it was her eating pattern that was almost certainly causing her headaches. Most nutritionists now consider three well-balanced meals a day is best as it evens out the energy supply, keeps hunger to a minimum and places less strain on the digestive system. Eating between meals with such foods as biscuits and chocolate is not good sense, as these are low in protein and vitamins, and result in a reduced appetite at meal-times. However, we do not live in a Utopian world, and I for one am rarely able to eat lunch. Of all the meals we eat, breakfast is the most neglected, usually from a lack of time or inclination, but as I have mentioned earlier it is the food we consume at breakfast that provides the basis of our energy for the coming day.

I could see that Norma was sceptical at the suggestion that missing breakfast was the cause of her migraine. Everyone needs energy to live, and this energy is mainly derived from sugar in the blood, which originates from food. As the sugar is used up, the amount available for energy decreases and hunger is experienced. If food is not eaten at this stage, the blood sugar will drop further and lassitude and headaches occur. Furthermore, as the brain becomes depleted of energy, blackouts and fainting can occur. Norma admitted that she had nearly passed out on several occasions but had attributed this to a direct effect of the migraine. By the morning, even if a large meal has been eaten the night before, the blood sugar level will be starting to fall too low so it is essential that it is replenished at breakfast. As Norma did not do this, by lunch-time her sugar had fallen low enough to produce her migraine attacks. It was important for her, therefore, to eat break-fast before starting work to raise her blood sugar level. If this reaches a normal level then energy is easily produced and there is a feeling of well-being.

Norma claimed that this could not be true as she always ate a chocolate bar at her break, which would surely produce a rise in her sugar level. This is excellent in theory but in practice it does not happen. When carbohydrate is eaten in the form of simple sugar, this does not need to be broken down by the stomach and can be absorbed straight into the bloodstream producing a rapid rise in blood sugar. This level is regulated by a substance called insulin and, if a lot of sugar reaches the blood at the same time, there is a corresponding surge in the production of insulin to ensure that the level of sugar does not go too high. The effect of this is to lower the blood sugar, but unfortunately the body is often so efficient that it overdoes things and too much insulin is formed too quickly. This excess then drops the blood sugar level far too low with the consequent lack of energy and fatigue.

Breakfast may therefore supply too little sugar to maintain

energy through the day or so much sugar that insulin is over-supplied. If breakfast consists mainly of cereals with sugar sprinkled on top, toast and marmalade, and tea or coffee with added sugar, then this will be absorbed very quickly. Research has clearly shown that the blood sugar level, although rising initially, will have fallen well below normal before lunch-time. The chocolate that Norma ate would have the same effect, as this is packed full of refined sugar. If carbohydrate is eaten as starch, however, this is absorbed more slowly and sugar only trickles into the bloodstream, giving a sustained pick-up hour after hour. This means that insulin is not overstimulated and energy is available throughout the day. Muesli, fresh fruit and eggs all supply starch to produce this effect.

The immune system is no different from any other part of the body in requiring energy to function efficiently, and if this is not available then it will quickly become ineffective with the subsequent drop in resistance to illness such as migraine. Norma's symptoms were therefore due partly to the direct effect of the low blood sugar and partly to the depressant effect it was having on her immune system. She was sceptical, however, that to cure her headaches all she had to do was to eat a healthy breakfast. To her credit, she agreed to try, and to her delight, her symptoms resolved within two weeks.

I have dwelt at some length on diet but I cannot stress too much how important it is to eat correctly. There is an old saying that 'we are what we eat'. Obviously this is an oversimplification, but the general principle is correct. What we eat and how we live are the two main causes of disease, and if these are inadequate then our immune system does not function effectively. We only have one life on this Earth and it is vital to make it a long and healthy one.

Summary of healthy diet
1) Balanced intake of carbohydrate and protein
2) Low fat intake — mainly unsaturated
3) Plenty of fresh fruit and vegetables
4) Supplement with minerals and vitamins
5) No additives

CHAPTER 4

Coping with stress

Stress is destructive as it suppresses the body's defence mechanism. Headaches can be the first sign of a depressed immune system, and if this is ignored it can lead to many serious illnesses including heart attacks, high blood pressure, and cancer. As more knowledge is gained, the damaging effects of stress become more and more apparent. If I had suggested to any of my patients five years ago that their health problems were the result of stress, they would have flatly denied it and moved to another doctor. However, attitudes have changed dramatically and many people are actively looking at ways of reducing their personal stress level.

Unfortunately, although most books and magazine articles recommend a stress-free existence, in practice this is not possible. Most of the events of a normal day impose some degree of stress upon us, quite apart from the occasional major disasters in our lives. It is our *response* that is critical, and we need to learn reactions that are positive and not harmful. Even if they were completely safe, there is no place for tranquillizers, as they merely treat the symptoms and not the cause. After a short time their effect wears off and it is necessary to increase the dose to notice any apparent benefit. This can ultimately lead to addiction.

Whilst most stress is harmful, some is actually beneficial, as illustrated by a patient whom I saw in the surgery last week. Gill R. is a 32-year-old woman who has had many problems including an unhappy marriage, a recent bereavement, and behavioural problems with her two young children. The continued stress and strain had taken a toll on her health and she had suffered with severe tension headaches for several months. There was no way that her situation could be significantly changed, as she wanted to keep the home together for the children's sake. I was fully expecting Gill to be in her usual unhappy state at her next appointment, but instead she was cheerful and lively. It transpired that a friend had persuaded her to go on a parachute jump and she had found the danger so stimulating that she had been on a 'high' for several days following the jump. There was no stopping Gill after that, and by the next time I saw her she had also started potholing, a sport she had wanted to do for years.

Both the activities that Gill had begun involved an element of danger, but she was stimulated by this stress rather than being depressed. The different response lies in the chemical reactions within the brain. If there is a desire to succeed in something that may seem difficult to achieve, e.g. winning a cup final, making a speech, or in Gill's case jumping from a plane, then the body responds by producing a substance called adrenaline. This has a tremendously stimulating effect and this effect can last for some time. However, if the stress is from a depressing or irritating situation then different chemicals, called steroids, are formed to help us overcome these difficulties. They are meant to be helpful but have damaging effects on our health if their level is kept high for too long, because they interfere with our immunity and other defence systems. It is this latter response that it is so important to control, as it is potentially damaging to our health. Gill had accomplished this by making her body produce so much adrenaline that this completely blocked out the production of any extra steroids. This is rather a drastic way of doing things and I am certainly not suggesting that you should start throwing yourself out of aeroplanes to combat day-to-day stress! What is required is a straightforward, practical plan to follow.

Dave H. came to see me suffering from severe migrainous headaches which he knew were caused by continuous stress. He could see himself eventually ending up in the local psychiatric hospital and asked me if there was a plan he could follow to help him. I reassured Dave that the greatest difficulty with stress is admitting to it: doing something about it is relatively easy.

Identifying stress

Step 1 is to go through a typical day identifying all the circumstances in which stress occurs and to see whether it can be reduced. Step 2 is then learning to cope with any stress that remains. By analysing our day we can see which situations will have a practical solution, those that will resolve themselves given time, and those that cannot be changed.

Dave was a 41-year-old accountant with three young children and a wife who worked mainly in the evenings running her own perfume business. As she was often very late to bed, Dave rose early each morning and made the children's breakfast and a cup of tea for his wife. His own breakfast was usually a piece of toast eaten hurriedly on the move and sometimes he didn't have anything. His youngest daughter was very active and noisy in the mornings and Dave found this irritating at a time when he was trying to collect his thoughts for the day ahead. As the children's school was on his direct route to work he would drop them off but if the traffic was heavy this would result in him being a few minutes late for his first appointment.

Dave had never really understood why he had studied account-ancy as he had absolutely no interest in the subject. He suspected that it had been his father's influence on him as it was the sort of safe job of which his father would have approved. To be fair, the pay was good and the job very secure, but there was little prospect of promotion. He would gladly have changed to something differ-ent but it would have meant a drop in income. This would have been difficult, as Dave was not a saver of money and with high mortgage repayments, the children's education, and ploughing money into his wife's business, a reduction in income would have been disastrous. Whilst he was not in severe debt, his credit card accounts were creeping up and the couple had stretched them-selves further with a car loan. He did supplement his income by writing articles for business magazines, but found he tended to try to do them late at night when he was very tired.

Dave had joined a local gym to keep fit but, with his wife work-ing in the evenings, he was forced to go at lunch-time. This tended to make his session rather hurried and meant he was not able to sit and relax during his break. When he returned home from work the children would leap upon him begging for a game of Monop-oly, and although he was longing for a rest, guilt would set in if he refused, so invariably they ended up playing. On one after-noon per week his work finished at 3 o'clock so he would collect the kids from school and cook the evening meal. By the time he had persuaded his son to do his homework and then had the usual argument over bedtimes, Dave was exhausted.

His marriage was a happy one, but for the past 18 months Dave had found a marked reduction in his sex drive and consequently the frequency of intercourse had drastically reduced. This had inevitably led to some tension in the marriage and it was a subject that Dave found extremely difficult to talk about. The added pressure had led to episodes of impotence with a marked drop in his self-confidence.

I have detailed this case as it is typical of many I see in the surgery. It is hardly surprising, when all the stressful factors of Dave's life are listed, that his immune system was suppressed and his migraine headaches had developed. It is amazing that many people do not appreciate how big a part negative stress plays in their lives until they list the causes as in this case.

When we analysed Dave's situation, it was clear that his lifestyle was beleaguered by a series of minor irritations from the start to the end of the day. It was important to sort out as many of these as possible before moving on to the causes of major stress. I advised him to set the alarm 15 minutes earlier to enable him to have an adequate and relaxing breakfast and to ask his wife if she would look after the children on some mornings, allowing Dave a quieter time before work. On the days when his wife had not worked the previous evening, Dave would be relieved from taking the children to school. Two days a week, the gymnasium was open at the end of working hours so his exercise could be taken at that time, and the habit of having to play with the children every night would be broken. These simple changes greatly improved Dave's enjoyment of life, and although it may sound as if I have been hard on his wife, in fact the changes made very little difference to her day.

The major causes of stress were his job, his financial situation, and his increasing impotence. It was virtually impossible for him to change his employment with his age against him and salary accounted for each month, so it was important for Dave to look at the positive aspects of his work rather than always being so negative. He was able to organize his workload virtually as he liked, was not constantly under supervision and, within reason, his hours were flexible. Alternatively, he could look for other outlets so that accountancy did not play such a major part in his life. As he was keen on writing and had already had several articles published, I advised him to broaden his field to include other areas of interest. The extra income from these articles would also allow him more freedom financially. Impotence is a complex problem and was certainly caused in Dave's case mainly by the dissatisfaction with his lifestyle. I urged him that it was vital to discuss the situation with his wife as in such cases this nearly always eases the tension for both partners.

I have not intended to give the impression that Dave would be able to lead a stress-free existence, but to show that a few simple modifications to his lifestyle would greatly reduce it. However, some stress is inevitable so the next step is to see how we can learn to live with it so it does not play a dominant or significant role in our lives.

Jean N. was a pleasant woman aged 38 who came to see me nearly at the end of her tether. She was recently divorced with two young children to bring up on her own and there was obviously no way that this could be done without a considerable degree of stress. Not only that, but everyone she met was always advising her on how to run her life and she was afraid to say anything to them for fear of hurting their feelings.

Jean had developed frontal headaches which were worse on waking and I was dismayed to notice on checking her blood pressure that it was considerably raised. This was in direct contrast to a reading twelve months previously when it had been perfectly normal, and I was sure it was the stress that had sent it up. It would have been a minor disaster to start her on drugs to lower it, so I formed a plan for her to cope with her stress.

Twelve-point plan for stress control

The key expression in stress control is positive thinking: can you really think yourself healthy? Research has shown that cheerful people are not as ill as those who are depressed. That does not mean they are not under stress, because everyone suffers from it, but they react in a positive manner. I'm sure you have at some time fought off a cold or flu because it has come at a time when you have been too busy to be ill. There are several ways of producing positive thought:

1) Look forward to something nice every day

I remember visiting an old farmer friend of mine in the early hours of one summer morning. His farm was high up in the hills and a considerable distance from my home. I was feeling a little grumpy at being called out, which must have showed on my face when I examined him, for he took me to his bedroom window and showed me the most beautiful sunrise I'd ever seen. 'Doctor,' he said, 'if nothing else pleasant happens to you today, at least you will have this memory to fall back on.' My irritation was lifted immediately and it gave me the stimulation to enjoy the coming day. The farmer died a week later, but his words have had a profound effect on my life. I am not fortunate enough to have a view like that in the morning, but I do make sure I have something pleasurable to look forward to every day. So many days are routine and uninteresting, especially in winter, that the negative side can soon take over. It doesn't have to be a major event — it can simply be relaxing with your favourite magazine, a visit to the hairdresser, a hot bath, an hour's yoga or keep fit, or an uninterrupted programme on television. Even if the rest of the day is disastrous, at least there will have been a period of positive pleasure during it. I emphasized to Jean, and to Dave in the previous case, that if I had to single out one factor alone to combat stress then this would be it.

2) Block negative thoughts before they start

Next time you have a problem, think about how you can improve the situation instead of dwelling on all the negative aspects. No one can feel on top of the world all the time, but if you force yourself to think and act positively then you will soon get into the habit of doing it naturally.

3) Don't hold back your feelings

Feeling angry but doing nothing about it is very negative and is a classic stress inducer. How many times have we all felt like saying something, but have stayed quiet and later regretted it? Whilst this stress will eat away at your immune system, acting in the opposite way has been shown to actually strengthen the body defences. The positive reaction is to release your tension and let the person know exactly how you feel. Next time you feel angry, let your feelings out. There's no need to over-react; just assert yourself calmly but firmly and you'll feel much better for it.

4) Don't let one bad event ruin your day or your life

An argument with a friend or relative doesn't mean that you don't get on with anyone. Everyone has differences of opinions but these are short-lived so try not to let them sour your day. Most of all, don't become negative and sulk or brood about things that have happened or look ahead to awful events that might occur.

5) Encourage yourself

If you do something well, give yourself a pat on the back and perhaps a reward like a glass of wine! If you are dressed for the evening and look in the mirror and think how smart you look, then go out with the knowledge that you will be the best there. The mind is very suggestive to ideas and if you keep telling yourself that you are the 'greatest' then you very soon will be!

6) Enjoy the first hour of the day

This is important as it sets the mood for the rest of the day. If you stay in bed even ten minutes too long it can produce a stressful time rushing around trying to dress, wash and eat breakfast all at the same time. Not only that, but if you have children they always choose that time to spill their cornflakes and mislay their school shoes! How much more relaxing to wake up half an hour earlier to a cup of tea courtesy of the teasmade at the bedside and to have a leisurely breakfast with the morning paper to browse through. Any problems will be easily dealt with and you can leave for work feeling calm and unruffled.

7) Plan the day ahead

The night before, write down everything to be done the following day. If there is far too much, then cross out what isn't strictly necessary and just do the rest. There is nothing worse than the feeling that there is too much that has to be done, and usually it means that very little is carried out properly. Naturally, try to ensure that you include everything you will actually enjoy doing.

8) Learn to delegate

This means both at home and at work. Don't fall into the trap of convincing yourself that if you don't do it then it won't be done properly. No one in this world is indispensable, so make sure your family and workmates realize that they cannot take advantage of you.

9) Learn to daydream

At different moments in your busy day, take some time out just to slow down and let your imagination take over. Picture yourself having fun, or relaxing, or taking part in some wild fantasy. The main point about daydreaming is that you are feeding your mind positive images which gives your immune system a regular boost.

10) Find an outlet for your stress

Try to find something that will help you unwind. It could be anything from squash to dancing as long as you find it rewarding. My own method is to go to a football match where I usually give vent to my stressful feelings by shouting at the referee!

11) Let yourself laugh

Laughing is therapeutic and an excellent medicine. It is not always easy to laugh to order, but if you smile frequently you can fool your body into feeling happy and a false smile will have the same effect as a natural one.

12) Sleep off your problems

While our bodies are at rest we go through a regenerative phase when body repairs are carried out. This is why spots and aches are often much improved after a night's sleep. Stress is similarly relieved, and we can often go to bed with a headache and find that it has disappeared by the morning. It is essential to give your body as much help as possible by having at least six to eight hours sleep per night.

Following these twelve steps in coping with stress is very simple and will produce dramatic results in a short time. There is nothing complicated about any of the stages and all that is required is a bit of extra effort. Both Jean and Dave followed this plan and their stress level is now much less and their headaches have virtually disappeared. Dave, however, still suffered from them at work and asked if there was anything further I could recommend. I reassured him that it is quite common for one stressful situation to persist, and at his age it is often associated with loss of interest and stimulation at work.

12 simple ways of coping with stress

1) Look forward to something nice each day
2) Block negative thoughts
3) Don't hold back your feelings
4) Don't let one bad day ruin your life
5) Encourage yourself
6) Enjoy the first hour of the day
7) Plan the day ahead
8) Learn to delegate
9) Learn to daydream
10) Find an outlet for your stress
11) Let yourself laugh
12) Sleep off your problems

I advised Dave that he should try to follow 'the three Cs' — commitment, control, and challenge. In fact, these can be applied to virtually any specific area of stress.

The three Cs

1) Commitment

This is actively involving yourself in whatever is happening around you. Instead of going to work thinking that it will be totally boring, try to be positive and more curious about the people with whom you work or come into contact. It is surprising that with only a small amount of extra commitment or imagination, the day can become less tedious.

2) Control

One of Dave's and Jean's problems was that they did not feel in control of their lives — in Dave's case particularly at work. Those who are well-endowed with this control factor believe and act as though they can influence the events happening around them by things they say and do. If you do not feel in control, then begin to start thinking that you *are*, in certain situations. Decide when something will take place, however mundane, and see that it is your decision which makes it do so. This could be as simple as making a cup of tea at a certain time or, in Dave's case, learning to keep a client waiting for a few minutes while he had a breather. If you *act* in control then you will *become* more in control of your life.

3) Challenge

To have an expectation that life will change, and that the changes which will take place will be exciting, is a great stimulus to your personal development. As Dave was an accountant, I advised him over a period of a few weeks to try to work out any possible diversification in his work to make it more interesting and challenging. Football was his main interest so he made enquiries at his local semi-professional club as to their needs for accountancy services, and they welcomed him with open arms. The work is stimulating and he has recently been made a director so he is also involved with the total running of the club. This was just the boost he needed and, strangely, now Dave has this new interest his job during the day does not seem so stressful.

Although we cannot avoid stress, we can all learn to live with it successfully rather than let it overwhelm us to the extent that it affects our mental and physical well-being. As there are enormous individual differences in the factors that cause us stress, and in our ability to cope, it is impossible in this chapter to provide the answer to everyone's problem. It should, however, have stimulated you to think about and identify the undesirable stresses in your life and thereby start to control them. We must aim to redress the balance between the stress which is exciting and positive, and that which is destructive and negative. Taking stock of ourselves from time to time can be an extremely beneficial exercise as many sources of unnecessary stress can be removed.

The people whose cases are described in this chapter all suffered severe problems with persistent headaches which were obviously directly related to stress. Once they had analysed themselves and taken simple steps both to reduce their stress level and to modify their reactions to it, their headaches quickly disappeared. There is no reason that, if you follow the same pathway, your own headaches should not do likewise.

CHAPTER 5

Exercise

Exercise has a major part to play in preventing and combating disease. Along with a stress-free lifestyle and a healthy diet, regular physical activity gives a tremendous boost to the immune system. It has been clearly shown that it produces a substantial increase in the number of T lymphocytes in the bloodstream and it is these that are so vital in keeping the body healthy. A depressed immune system will allow most types of headache to develop, so it is important to take every available step to stimulate it.

Walking

A classic example was Alan P., a 57-year-old patient who came to my consulting room complaining of quite severe muscular headaches which gradually worsened during the day. Alan was a jeweller by trade and over the years had built up his own business which was very successful. He was not under stress, and he ate a wholefood diet, but he never took any exercise. Having many valued customers, he liked to be always available for them so he never left the shop during the day. I made the obvious suggestion to him that he should go for a regular walk for about twenty minutes at lunch-time and see if it would ease his problem. It did not surprise me to find that his headaches cleared completely.

Most situations are not as simple or clear-cut as this but it is amazing how easily exercise can be excluded from our lives. I am not talking just about actual sports, but equally about exercise in our home and working environment. A hundred years ago we were much more physically active: many people lived in rural areas, and walking was their only form of transport. With scientific development we now can live comfortably with the minimum of effort. The motor car takes us to the shops where lifts and escalators save us climbing stairs. Indeed, as technology develops, it will not be long before we can order our shopping without even going to the supermarket. At home, washing machines, dishwashers and vacuum cleaners pander to our needs and there are even food processors and electric knives to save us from slicing the vegetables and carving the meat! Exercise-saving devices have now reached such extremes that we can alter the channel on our television set without rising from our chair. I would not wish to labour the point, but it has recently been calculated that the average adult in the UK will spend about 15 years of their life sitting in front of the television. Outside the home, there is now the powered lawn-mower, and firewood need not be chopped, as most people have gas or electric fires. Sport has not entirely escaped the exercise-saving trend, as golf can be played without having to walk between shots. In Alan's case, described above, his body was crying out for some exercise and it did not take much effort on his part to realize the benefit. How unfortunate it is that society is engaged, with all these inventions, in ensuring that we perform less and less.

Swimming

So why is it that we allow this to happen? I remember talking at great length to a 63-year-old patient, Emily D., who was suffering from a combination of tension and sinus headaches. She had already improved her diet, but took very little exercise other than to walk to the corner shop for her groceries. Some people have never been actively inclined, but Emily had in fact played in the school netball and tennis teams and represented the county at gymnastics. On leaving school, however, she had to work hard in the local factory to bring extra money into the home so had little time for exercising. By the time things improved financially, the incentive to carry on with her sport had been lost and was never regained.

The problem in Emily's situation was that when she was at

school all the games were competitive and it would have been more beneficial to introduce her to some recreational pursuits that would have been useful in later life. In the long term, the ideal sports to maintain health and fitness involve regular rhythmic contractions of the large muscle groups. Thus Emily's netball and tennis could have been combined with activities such as hiking, swimming and cycling. These have the advantage that they can be played either on a competitive basis or just for fun and do not require a team or partner to perform them.

The crisis times for giving up or continuing sporting activities are classically on leaving school, at 30 years old, and in middle age. As described above, the change from competitive to non-competitive recreation is a major landmark, and the age of 30 is often the age when there is a feeling that 'I cannot keep up with the younger ones and don't want to be another also-ran'. This attitude can lead to a complete cessation of exercise. For the first 25 years of our lives we try to speed ourselves up, and after that we do everything possible to slow down. At 40 years old or middle age is when the excuse of 'I'm not as young as I used to be' is put forward for backing out of anything physical. This drift into a society that worships television, motor cars and fast food has led to a severe drop in overall fitness with the consequent development of all kinds of illness including headaches.

Emily understood all this in principle but could not really appreciate why exercise would be beneficial to her now that she was reaching her later years. I explained to her that ageing is a natural process which cannot be stopped, but there is increasing evidence that it can be slowed down by regular physical activity. This means that she would never appear old or beyond her years. Her mind would remain fresh and attentive and her body would stay lean and alert with good muscle tone. The heart and lungs would develop plenty of spare capacity and she herself would feel much younger. Her immune system would be strengthened and resistance to illness fortified, thus eradicating her troublesome headaches.

This was all very well in theory but to someone like Emily, who was used to a quiet home life with only a short walk to the local shop each day, it seemed beyond her reach. I pointed out to her that she lived just around the corner from the town's leisure centre and there were plenty of activities that were organized for people in exactly her situation. On Thursday mornings there was free admission to the swimming pool for pensioners, and on other days of the week there were keep fit and yoga classes that she could join. Naturally, as Emily had been on her own for some time she was a little reluctant to join these activities but I was able to introduce her to one of the course organizers who reassured her that there were many people in the same position. You can imagine how surprised I was about six weeks later when, struggling up the pool using my own laboured version of breast-stroke, I was passed by Emily doing a perfect back-stroke. We had a coffee together after the swim and I was amazed at the change in her appearance. Gone was the negativity of a short time previously and it had been replaced by someone with energy and vitality. Never had she felt better, and of course her headaches were no longer any problem.

It is not difficult to produce a convincing case for regular exercise, and most people will accept that it is beneficial to their health. So many patients who complain of headaches lead a sedentary life, but it can be difficult to know how to start exercising and what form it should take. Whilst it is impossible to describe all the different types of sporting activities, I have tried in the next two cases to illustrate a typical approach.

Mike S. was a 40-year-old man who ran a newspaper wholesale business, which was mainly night work. Over the years he had managed on a few hours' sleep each morning before going to the pub for a pint at lunch-time. He smoked 20 cigarettes a day and was overweight. Mike had recently developed migraine headaches on the left side behind the eye and he had the insight to realize that it was probably his lifestyle that was at fault. He stopped smoking, changed his diet and came to seek advice as he wanted to replace his daily trip to the 'Golden Bear' with some form of exercise. He did not particularly want to take up a competitive sport, mainly because he did not have anyone to play with, and, as he worked irregular hours, he preferred some activity he could do on his own.

Mike had led this unhealthy way of life since leaving school over 20 years previously and therefore it was important that he did not attempt to correct this immediately. There is no way that 20 years of soft living could be lost in the first 30 minutes' exercise. Mike was keen to start, having bought a new tracksuit and running shoes, but I stressed to him that he could not simply leave the world of beer and cigarettes behind and head for the hills! Firstly, as he was so unfit, it was more likely that the slightest incline would be too much for him, leading to total demoralization. Many people give up after the first attempt as they feel a failure, which is a shame as everyone needs a gradual approach. The other problem with sudden exertion is that it can produce a severe strain on the heart. Like the immune system, the heart thrives on exercise but this must be built up by degrees.

Circuit training

Ideally, the place to start is at the local gymnasium, as this has the advantage of being supervised and a circuit can be worked out for each individual. If general improvement in fitness is needed, as in Mike's case, then a programme for both the upper and lower body can be devised. Nowadays gyms do not consist only of weights — the equipment is much more sophisticated and can pick out individual muscle groups. There is, for example, an apparatus purely for the hamstrings at the back of the legs and one for the shoulder muscles. Electric power joggers, which are like moving conveyor belts, now mean that distances can be run in the gym without the potential embarrassment of being seen in an exhausted state by the neighbours. As fitness develops, the instructor will gradually increase the severity of the circuit.

Mike did very well with these exercises, but there were times when he felt he needed to be in the fresh air, and as he was by now considerably fitter, he asked what I thought he should try next.

Jogging

Jogging is ideal for many people as basically you can run anywhere at any time provided that the surface is good and, if it is winter, that the area is adequately lit. There is a certain thrill at donning a pair of running shorts and shoes and jogging along the pathways of a local beauty spot. In the case of a job that involves travelling, then nothing could be easier than to take your trainers with you. This form of exercise has the added advantage of being relatively inexpensive as the only outlay is on shoes and clothing.

I advised Mike to start with a simple jog of about a mile and to ensure that it ended back at his house. When he was comfortable at this distance he could then increase it in stages. Some athletes are able to run many miles at a time but to lesser mortals a maximum of three to four miles is ideal. Mike had the advantage of being able to train at quiet times of the day, as running in rush hour traffic with all the fumes will merely raise the level of carbon monoxide in the blood. This in itself can produce severe headaches. Running when tired late in the day is also not to be recommended and no one should ever take any exercise when suffering from a cold as the virus can spread to affect the heart muscle.

Cycling

Mike had a yen to try cycling as he had enjoyed this at school and I assured him that this is a superb form of exercise. Top-class cyclists are probably the fittest athletes in the world as regards both their immune systems and their hearts. It can be made either difficult or easy and can be done individually or in a group. There are few pleasanter ways of taking exercise than spinning along quiet country lanes on a balmy summer evening. Whether you ride for ten or a hundred miles, it is an enjoyable form of exercise as it is always varied and never boring. The only real drawback is that many roads are not suitable for cycling, because of volume of traffic and the lack of consideration for the cyclist from the average motorist. An exercise bicycle may be the answer, but this lacks the fun of the outdoor life and pedalling in the same place for 30 minutes is very boring. This tedium can be offset by watching the television or talking to someone, but somehow it can never replace the real thing. I advised Mike, as with his jogging, to build up gradually — perhaps only a couple of miles to start with — and again to make sure that he ended up back at home and not somewhere in the wilds. A comfortable saddle sounds obvious, but I have found to my cost that the new racing saddles which are very narrow and hard create severe discomfort in the buttock region.

In bad weather, I would recommend swimming to everyone, as this is something that uses almost every major muscle group in the body. In addition, since the body weight is adequately supported, it is ideal for those individuals who have problems with obesity or who suffer from arthritis. Mike said he would try this as it was something in which he could involve other members of his family. Most people were taught to swim as children and, like cycling, once learned it is never forgotten. However, if you cannot swim it is never too late to learn, and once you overcome that initial self-consciousness you will come to enjoy it. The only disadvantage of swimming is finding a pool that is not so crowded, particularly at weekends and school holidays, that good quality swimming becomes extremely difficult. Many leisure centres, however, do have time set aside for lane swimming only.

Mike thus had his exercise programme set out for him. His basic routine was circuit training at the gym. On some days he would replace one of these sessions with a two to three mile jog. On summer days, or if he was feeling particularly energetic, he would go for a cycle ride, and in bad weather or with the family he would turn to swimming. These are all excellent forms of exercise for boosting the immune system and in general are the easiest to initiate. The combination is to be recommended as it reduces boredom and thus increases compliance. The question that Mike and many others often ask is: how much exercise should we actually do?

Research has shown that three sessions of 20–30 minutes per week are quite sufficient to keep the body fit and healthy. This applies both to the immune system and to the heart, which also benefits greatly from exercise. However, there is an obvious problem here, as 30 lengths of hard swimming requires much more effort than walking for a similar time. There is a simple calculation that can be made as a guide to the intensity of exercise needed, based on the pulse rate. This can be counted, when resting, at the wrist and is always expressed as beats per minute. In Mike's case his rate was 68 beats per minute but a normal range can vary between 35 and 90. When you are exercising, the heart speeds up so as to pump more blood into the muscles, but whilst the heart thrives on exercise, it is important that it is not put under too much strain. A simple guide is to subtract one's age from 220 and this gives the maximum rate that the heart can beat. So for Mike this was 220 minus 40 = 180, but for a 20-year-old it would be 220 minus 20 = 200, and for someone of 65 it would be 220 minus

65 = 155 (see Table 1). For the most benefit from exercise, the heart rate should be maintained at about 75 per cent of this figure, so the heart is having to work harder but there is still plenty in reserve. So at 20 years old the rate would be 150; at 40, as in Mike's case, it would be 135; and at 65 it would be 116. This sounds complicated, but in practice it is very simple: the pulse is counted at some stage of the activity and this will show whether these beneficial heart rates are being achieved. If we use Mike as an example, when he was swimming, his rate was only 110 beats per minute so he increased his effort in the pool, but when he was running, his rate reached 165 so he knew he was overdoing it and slowed down.

Table 1: Guide to heart rate during exercise

Age	Maximum heart rate	Heart rate for maximum benefit
20	220	150
30	190	144
40	180	135
50	170	127
60	160	120
70	150	112

Simple rule of thumb:
220 minus age = max rate minus 25% = maximum benefit.

Not everyone is prepared to take exercise this seriously, and it is certainly true that plenty of people become very fit without the aid of pulse measurements. Anne C. was a 64-year-old pensioner whose husband had also recently retired. She was complaining of crushing-type headaches which had started a few months before her leaving party at work. These were obviously muscular from the associated tension.

I asked Anne how she intended to spend her retirement and she replied that both she and her husband wanted to spend more time in the fresh air. They both asked me whether it would be beneficial for them to cycle as they were totally fed-up with driving and other motorists. I was full of enthusiasm and this encouragement led to them going out and buying a pair of folding bicycles. Neither of them had ridden for 30 years, and starting to ride a bike again after three decades of easy living is not without its problems. As you become older something seems to happen to your sense of balance and they both found that, when they glanced behind to see whether any cars were coming, the bikes would wobble! However, they both overcame these early setbacks and now lead an active and enjoyable life. They are slow compared with the 'shorts and singlets set' but their enthusiasm is undaunted and Anne's headaches have disappeared completely. There is a message here, not only for the desk-bound types but for the not-so-young and not-so-fit people still at work to buy a bike and take to the highways and byways.

Usually the best form of exercise is the type you enjoy the most. Nora H. was a 52-year-old whom I had advised to take up some form of exercise to build up her immune system. This I hoped would cure her migraine and also relieve her stressful feelings. I suggested walking, cycling or swimming but she was not keen and asked whether dancing would be too strenuous. I reassured her that the body was made to dance; just think how easily you sway to music or tap your feet to beat out a rhythm. The first thing that small children do is to wiggle their hips and move their legs when they hear a tune. Sadly, in later life many people do not dance because they are embarrassed and self-conscious. Nora joined the local class advertising lessons in ballroom dancing, which she had always enjoyed. To bring her exercise level up further she also had a tap dancing lesson every Thursday.

Dancing

As I personally knew very little about dancing, Nora took me along one day to show me how strenuous it can be, and if anyone thinks that ballroom dancing is reserved for the older generation then think again. The age range at that particular class was from 20 to 80. Seeing everyone swirling vigorously around the floor away from the stresses of life was most stimulating. As the dancers came off the floor there were beads of sweat on their brows but smiles of enjoyment on their faces.

The important point about dancing is that you can slow it down or speed it up depending on how you feel. This is especially true with tap dancing where each step is learnt very slowly, then the music is gradually speeded up. In other words it is a graded form of exercise. Anyone can take up dancing as all you need is a pair of shoes and plenty of enthusiasm. I have included this case because the exercise and enjoyment improved Nora's quality of life, and the boost to her immune system cleared her headaches. I have now firmly added dancing to the list of possible activities I recommend.

With the cases illustrated above I have tried to show that there is a wide range of sports available that are beneficial. The only one I have reservations about is squash, as this is a particularly strenuous form of exertion. Severe strain can be put on the heart to try to meet the sudden extra demands placed on the circulation. This is acceptable if the players are already very fit, but it is not to be recommended to anyone just taking up sport, or indeed to anyone who only plays squash occasionally. It is interesting to note that headaches can actually be caused by such demanding exercise and several of my patients have complained that their migraine attacks have started on the squash court.

Our modern-day lack of physical exertion and the large amount of leisure time available make a decision necessary as to whether some of that time should be used to improve the body's fitness. It is sad that most of us choose to avoid sport of any kind. Yet there are signs that increasing numbers of people are recognizing that health is their own responsibility and that regular moderate exercise can do much to preserve well-being and provide an excellent quality of life. Headaches — from whatever cause — can disappear like magic, even if they are longstanding.

In this section I have tried to emphasize that a combination of stress control, a wholefood diet and regular exercise will so increase the efficiency of the immune system that it will cure over 90 per cent of headaches without any further measures. However, there are some headaches that are stubborn, and it may be necessary to try more complex measures and in some instances to seek professional help. In the following chapters I have detailed the approach and treatment to each individual type of headache and the alternative therapies that should be considered.

Most important of all is to avoid taking drugs, as these merely suppress the symptoms without treating the underlying causes.

Indeed, most drugs actually have a depressant effect on the immune system. Your own immune system is your most vital weapon in your bid to reach optimum health and you owe it to yourself to maintain it in perfect condition. No one should settle for anything less.

Curing your headaches

CHAPTER 6

Muscular headaches

To feel the lifting of a crushing weight on the top of the head or the easing of a tight band around the scalp is a wonderful experience. Unfortunately, this relief is often short-lived and the headache usually returns. Tension is an important factor in this type of headache — this is not just the sensation of feeling tense but actual tightness in the muscles as well. At the same time as affecting the muscles of the scalp producing severe headaches, this tension will also be present to a lesser extent in muscles in other parts of the body. If you keep the immune system in peak condition as outlined in the previous three chapters, these headaches will usually not develop. However, this may involve a major change in lifestyle and therefore will take some time to achieve. Not only that, but there are bound to be times in our lives when we are under stress, when our diet slips and when the thought of an early morning jog holds little appeal. To cure these headaches, therapy must produce a release of the muscular tension that is producing them and there are several ways that this can be accomplished.

These techniques are well illustrated by the case of Tina A., who was a 35-year-old with quite severe and persistent tension headaches. Her previous work had been as a secretary but she had given this up to bring up her two children. They were both now at school and Tina, feeling that she needed more of a challenge, had started her own business which involved grooming company sales teams in their dress and appearance. This business had the added advantage that it could be run from home and therefore she was usually there when the children came home from school. However, as with any new business, it required a fair amount of investment and after a year the money coming in was just about equal to the outgoings. Family finances were already very stretched and Tina was under enormous stress trying to make her business work profitably.

Her diet had always been excellent and regular yoga classes each week kept her physically fit. As a family they had many different activities so her life did not lack excitement. The stress therefore was the main problem and Tina well appreciated this, but there did not seem to be an easy answer. If she gave up her business and went out to work then her financial problems would disappear. However, Tina was determined not to follow this line and believed that, given time, her business would become profitable. Until then she had to find a way to cope with her headaches which, as well as being very painful, were knocking the edge off her work. As tension was the main feature, the use of one of the relaxation techniques would certainly help if not cure the headaches.

Breathing

I explained to Tina that our breathing is of vital importance and that we breathe in different ways according to our needs at that particular time. When asleep our breathing is deep and slow but when under pressure it becomes shallow and fast with only the top half of the lungs fully expanded. When we are angry the pattern is rapid and irregular, but if we relax it becomes gentle, rhythmic and very quiet. So the way we breathe alters our consciousness from stressed to relaxed and from relaxed to sleep. By deliberately controlling our breathing, we can steady the system, stop panic from mounting or deal with a difficult situation. It will reduce pressure and enable us to keep cool and clear-headed throughout the day. Tina was most interested in this as she had noticed that she always tended to overbreathe when under stress. Not only that, but her headaches always seemed to occur at times of panic as to whether her business was really going to be successful.

The method is simple to learn. Firstly, sit back comfortably in a chair — it is not necessary to lie down. Allow your shoulders to droop and take five slow deep breaths in and out. Having done this, you are now ready to start the relaxing phase of the breathing. Take a first deep breath in and now breathe out fully as if you were a balloon deflating completely. Go down yourself with the deflating balloon and allow your lungs to refill without any effort on your part. This is because you are primarily concerned with deflating yourself and driving out all the stress and tension with the exhaled air. As you repeat this cycle you will feel yourself becoming more floppy with each deflating breath. As more of your body goes limp, and the irritation and tension disappear, your head will become clearer and clearer. After only two to three minutes you can take a deep energizing breath, feel alert and start to breathe away quietly and normally. I often practise this method during a busy surgery, between patients, as it only takes a couple of minutes. I advised Tina that this is a useful tension reducer in the middle of a harassing day, or when everything begins to pile up on top of her.

Relaxation

While the control of breathing is a useful quick method of calming tension in difficult situations, it may be necessary with more severe headaches to learn a method for relaxing the whole body. This does require some time commitment, in the region of 10–15 minutes twice a day, but with practice this will be reduced and the benefit will be felt for longer.

There are many different ways of performing relaxation exercises, some of which seem totally incomprehensible. I have therefore evolved two methods that are simple to follow.

Method A

Lie flat on your back, with a pillow or cushion under the back of your head — this keeps the spine and neck straight during the relaxation. Next draw your knees up so they are bent but comfortable: quite often it is useful to put a cushion under them as support. Close your eyes and take slow, regular breaths in and out through your nose. Continue with this slow, regular breathing for 3–4 minutes, as this is relaxing in itself.

Then make a conscious effort to relax your muscles. Start with your feet and gradually work up your body until you finish with your head and neck. It is actually easier to relax muscles by tensing them first and then releasing them. So as an example you would start by tensing the muscles in your toes and relaxing them, then your calf muscles, then your knees, thighs and so on. With tension headaches you will find that the muscles in the scalp may be stubbornly reluctant to relax and a little extra effort is needed for this area. Carry on for a total of 15 minutes and then gradually straighten your legs and sit up slowly.

Method B

Sit upright in a chair, preferably one with a firm back, with your feet flat on the floor in a comfortable position. Sit in a relaxed upright posture, ensuring that your neck and spine are straight, but without straining. Your hands should be resting in your lap. As in the previous exercise, close your eyes and start slow, regular, comfortable breathing. Continue doing this for 3–4 minutes and then concentrate on first tensing and then relaxing your muscles, starting with your feet and working your way up the body. The whole exercise, as with the first one, should take about 15 minutes. I explained to Tina that this is particularly useful as it can be used while sitting at a desk or typewriter. Relaxation and therefore relief of headaches can be achieved very rapidly even under these conditions.

Tension headaches usually increase in severity throughout the day and Tina was finding that by night time they were so intense that they were keeping her awake. As sleep will normally relieve these headaches, it is vital for all sufferers to have sufficient, and often a short nap in the day is beneficial. There is a simple technique which I taught Tina to use to achieve this: start by taking a deep breath in, very slowly feeling the breath fill up your chest until it reaches the mouth. As you breathe out, imagine yourself blowing the breath out of your mouth then round in a circle and back through an imaginary hole in your stomach. Then, as you breathe in again, the air is drawn up through the chest to the mouth, out and down to the stomach and then up through the chest again. The rhythm must be slow and feel comfortable. The most important part of this procedure is the full involvement of the mind in the circular process of breathing. Keep a mental picture in your mind and follow it round at all times making sure that the mind thinks only of this circular rhythm. I often use this method myself, and rarely have to take more than a dozen breaths to succeed. You will find that your eyes will automatically follow the circle from the mouth, down to the stomach and in again. Should you wake in the night then you will quickly be able to fall asleep again.

Tina was a particularly good subject and the relaxation techniques worked extremely well, to the extent that when her headaches started she was easily able to settle them. In fact, when she started using regular relaxation most days, her level of tension dropped and her tendency to develop headaches virtually disappeared.

I have taught many patients the art of relaxation but have found occasionally that they find it difficult to do on their own. For this reason I have a collection of relaxation tapes which take you through the various methods of relieving tension. There is a wide variety of these cassettes, to suit different situations, for example there is one to make you feel energetic in the morning and another to help you to sleep at night. They are set to soothing music or spoken in a calming voice.

Active relaxation

For some people the use of a more active form of relaxation is most beneficial. I am sure you have found that taking a brisk walk can often induce a feeling of well-being and an easing of tension. When I was at college studying for exams, by playing football twice a week I was able to relieve my stress and for two or three hours to put work out of my mind completely. Different activities suit different people, but one I would particularly recommend is yoga. By practising methods of moving, stretching and breathing which came into being thousands of years ago, it is possible to eradicate aches and pains, create suppleness and energy, and even delay signs of ageing! Yoga movements are an excellent preventive measure, and ten minutes each day will increase life and energy flow to each part of the body, preventing the rigidity that leads to tension.

Rose T. was a 53-year-old woman who had suffered with tension headaches for many years and was desperate to find a way to relieve them. There was no specific cause, and she was not keen to simply relax at home. Rose was a little put off when I suggested yoga, fearing that strange religious beliefs would be imposed on her, but I was able to reassure her that nothing was further from the truth. The best way of practising yoga is to use a combination of a once- or twice-weekly class plus daily usage at home. The trouble of only practising it at home is that you may develop bad habits without anyone there to correct them. Not only that, but going out to group yoga is often beneficial in itself. There is usually a course at your local leisure centre, or if not they will certainly be able to recommend one. It really led to an upturn in Rose's life as she is now more relaxed but more energetic at the same time and her tension headaches have been relieved for the first time in years.

Massaging the scalp

With severe muscular headaches, it may be possible to relieve the tension by massaging the scalp to relieve the muscle spasm. Connie F. was a 63-year-old who had perfected this technique and one day in the surgery she taught it to me. It is in three parts:

1) Close your eyes, take a deep breath in and release your jaw. Place both hands at the centre of your forehead just above the eyebrows and stroke firmly outwards. Move up the forehead in three stages and repeat several times.

2) Keeping your eyes closed, take a few more deep breaths. Place your middle fingers at the upper corner of each eye, just beneath the eyebrow. Press firmly inwards for a count of five and then release. Repeat this by pressing all the way along the brow bone to the outer corner and then continue underneath the eye.

3) Massage the scalp with both hands, working firmly backwards from the crown of the head.

This massage is remarkably simple to perform and most effective at relieving the distress of tension headaches.

The methods of controlling tension headaches described above, using breathing control, relaxation, scalp massage and active relief of tension, are simple to learn and can be carried out easily at home or at work. In this book, however, I want to cover the full range of therapies available, and just occasionally I come across patients who are unable to cure their headaches themselves and need the help of a professional.

Mary H. was a 39-year-old housewife with crippling headaches which were so bad that she found it difficult to sit and relax. Her mind would keep wandering back to her pain and it seemed that nothing would relieve it. They had started as a result of her husband losing his job with the consequent financial problems. He had become very negative and lost all belief in himself, so it threw an extra burden on Mary to keep the family together. She did not want the children to suffer so took on extra work herself, which further deepened her husband's lack of confidence and increased the friction at home. Mary found that trying to relax on her own was impossible, partly because her problems seemed to have no solution, and also because the atmosphere in the house was not conducive to it. Her visit to the surgery was really a last resort in the hope that I could suggest some method of at least helping her to cope.

Biofeedback

I explained to Mary that there was a special form of therapy available which enables the person to become aware of the functioning of a particular part of the body. Once they have been taught this, they are then trained to alter the activity of whichever part is causing the trouble. In Mary's case it was the muscles of the scalp that were producing the headaches so this was the area on which the treatment would focus. About ten years ago, biofeedback was the fashionable form of treatment for a wide range of illnesses. In the intervening years careful research has shown that while there are limitations to its use, it is extremely effective in a small number of conditions. Fortunately, tension headaches are particularly suitable and Mary was very keen to try it out. It may sound complicated, but in practice it is very simple.

First the patient is attached to a machine that records activity in the muscles around the scalp. This activity is represented by means of a flashing light or a beeping sound. It is known that anyone with chronic headaches has increased tension in these muscles and so at the beginning of the session there are almost continuous sounds or flashing lights. As the muscles become more relaxed the lights or sounds start to reduce in intensity and this continues as each treatment session produces more and more easing of the muscle tension. The main benefit is that it produces a controlled state of relaxation which is particularly focused on a specific area of the body. Some therapists believe that it is possible to learn this form of treatment without the use of machines but I have not found this to be true. With the use of flashing lights it is easy to see how modifying your actions to lessen the degree of tension will produce a positive effect. This immediately induces a feeling of confidence in the patient that the treatment is working.

Counselling

Mary did exceptionally well with the biofeedback and her headaches greatly diminished. Most of the time they were insignificant but they still tended to occur at times, especially when she was feeling irritated by her husband's negative approach to his situation. Mary had a great deal of sympathy for him and could not really understand why she should feel so angry. In my practice, as well as in many others, we now employ a counsellor who is trained to deal with these sorts of circumstances. Counselling is a process whereby the person concerned can learn to manage the emotional and practical realities that face them. Since almost anyone can set up as a counsellor, it is wise to ensure before starting that she or he is qualified and experienced. Your own doctor will normally be able to advise you or, failing that, one of the self-help agencies. There are many different techniques, but to be successful the counsellor must be warm and understanding.

Mary visited the counsellor at my own practice twice a week for a month and the therapy was based on two approaches: firstly, reassurance, which is the most widely used form of counselling. Bland reassurance just for the sake of it is seldom useful, but careful listening will help identify the main stress and then positive information can be put in a form which is easy to understand and remember. The second approach, which is usually more beneficial, is behavioural counselling. This is aimed at relieving a specific difficulty by studying the patterns of behaviour that led up to it. The response to the situation can then be modified by learning more useful ways of dealing with it. In Mary's situation it was her feelings towards her husband that were the problem, as she was unable to accept his negativity towards himself, although she felt that she should be sympathetic because he had lost his job. These feelings were producing continuing stress and leading to the tension headaches. The counsellor was able to show Mary that by unintentionally being critical of her husband, she was making him react against her. When she modified her approach and became more supportive, her husband became much more positive and was soon back in full-time employment.

Obviously, this is an oversimplification, but it is surprising how, when you discuss problems with a trained counsellor, he or she will usually see a beneficial line of approach to a troublesome situation. Of course, I am not saying that Mary's husband was not at fault, because he undoubtedly was, but it is unusual for both partners to agree to be seen together so we only had Mary to work with. Once Mary's worries were eased, the tension in her scalp muscles relaxed and her headaches disappeared.

Homoeopathic treatment

Nowhere in this chapter have I recommended the use of drug therapy in the treatment of tension headaches. I don't really think anyone would argue with the use of the occasional paracetamol, but they should be avoided for long-term use because of potential side-effects. Headaches caused by stress do tend to be recurrent, and I am often asked whether there is anything that can be taken for them. Homoeopathic remedies are particularly effective and are free of adverse effects. They can be used for several kinds of headaches, so to avoid repetition I have described the principles of homoeopathy in Chapter 11. For the remedies to work to maximum benefit, it is preferable to consult a registered homoeopath, but there are some general guidelines that can be followed. There are three effective preparations for muscular headaches, depending on the type of person you are, and these can be obtained from all health food shops.

1) Gelsemium

This is particularly useful for the kind of tension headaches that are tight, like a weight crushing down on the head. The symptoms invariably start around 10 o'clock in the morning and progressively worsen through the day. Damp, close weather exacerbates them, and there is often associated muscle aching in other parts of the body.

2) Glonoine

Headaches that feel as if the head is going to burst respond well to glonoine. There is usually a violent pounding of the head in time with the pulse, and heat or the sun make them worse.

3) China Sulph.

This is used for headaches that start in the back of the neck and spread rapidly over the whole head, which feels sweaty and damp. The pain is worsened by being in a stuffy atmosphere and by bending down or turning the head and eyes. The person often feels nauseated, but still wants to eat.

Tension headaches continue to be a scourge for millions throughout the world. However, relief is largely in our own hands and if you adopt one or more of the remedies described in this chapter then you will be able to eliminate them and lead a happier and healthier life.

Methods of relieving tension headaches
1) Breathing control
2) Relaxation
3) Scalp massage
4) Active relaxation
5) Biofeedback
6) Counselling
7) Homoeopathy

CHAPTER 7

Migraine

Migraine is a most miserable condition which can completely destroy the quality of life. If approached in the right way, however, it can be beaten, although sufferers will quickly discover that everyone is a self-appointed authority on its cause and cure. The one thing you will probably not find is sympathy and understanding, except from others similarly afflicted. Employers often think that attacks of migraine are merely a convenient excuse to avoid unpleasant situations at work.

Unfortunately, some people pretend that they have migraine and do not hesitate to use it to avoid social functions or work, much to the detriment of genuine sufferers. These same people are also the ones who are frequently cured by whatever treatment is currently enjoying popularity. This raises false hopes and despair in the severely disabled patient who wastes time and money on unproven and usually ineffectual treatment. A classical migraine attack is easy to diagnose although the nature of the headache may vary and there may be two or three kinds which occur under different conditions.

One afternoon I was called to see Jackie Y., a 40-year-old receptionist, who gave a typical history. For some hours before the attack she felt edgy and generally unwell, and then developed flashing lights, loss of part of her field of vision and a severe one-sided headache with nausea and vomiting. These features alone are sufficient to diagnose migraine, but Jackie said that often the headache was more general or occasionally the pain was localized around one eye. It is this variation in presentation that often leads to a delay in the correct diagnosis. The most reliable symptom, if there is any doubt, is a deep boring sensation in one or other eye accompanied by nausea and Jackie often experienced this at work without developing a full-blown attack. Her discomfort was strikingly aggravated by bright lights, particularly strip-lights, and by bending, coughing and straining. No one seemed to appreciate the intensity of the pain, which was often of unbearable severity and when each attack was over she would have a generally washed-out feeling for several days. Drug therapy had proved of little value and Jackie's only relief was to go to bed and try to sleep. Her social life was ruined, and she had already lost two jobs from taking so much time off work.

The first step on the road to a cure was to plot the pattern of Jackie's headaches for, while migraine can occur randomly, there are usually some common triggering factors. By analysing her lifestyle we were able to identify several features that are common to many people.

In women, a pattern associated with the menstrual cycle is frequent, with attacks occurring in the days before or at the onset of a period. Jackie had been on the pill, which had precipitated her headaches, and this had to be withdrawn. When she was pregnant her attacks had cleared completely, although this is impractical as a long-term solution!

There was a weekend pattern, with episodes occurring on waking on Saturday and Sunday. She had plenty of other episodes at random on other days but the weekends were constant. Prolonged deep sleep is a well-known precipitant in migraine and Jackie looked glum at the thought of foregoing her lie-in on these days. Fortunately, all that is needed is to arrange to wake at the normal time, get up for a few minutes and then return to bed and sleep. This is a simple common-sense manoeuvre which is nearly always successful.

Sunlight may be a hazard and some patients dread summer holidays. Summer sunshine on wet roads and misty early morning sun in winter are often cited particularly by car drivers and should be avoided. Dark glasses must be worn as a preventive measure.

There may be a seasonal variation, and certainly cases increase at Christmas and New Year as most sufferers notice a tendency for alcohol to provoke attacks. With excess food intake at the festive season there may be a rebound lowering of blood sugar between meals which can bring on a migraine headache. I stressed to Jackie the importance of moderation at this time.

At some stage a bad run of headaches will occur which usually start as a dull muzzy feeling and build up into more typical migraine headaches. These serial attacks often follow periods of prolonged stress and the person may suspect that they have a brain tumour.

Strenuous physical exertion is a well-known cause of migraine and this can be added to the catalogue of jogging-induced health problems. Jackie often experienced attacks after a game of squash, but we were able to prevent these with the use of homoeo- pathic tablets taken before the game.

By far the commonest trigger is food, and there are undoubtedly many people who cease to have migraine attacks if they exclude certain foodstuffs from their diets. This is well illustrated by the case of Lorna I., a 34-year-old shop assistant who suffered from severe migraine associated with vomiting in the week before her period. The major difficulty was that from her first symptom to a full-blown headache only took ten minutes. Lorna realized that the majority of her attacks started just after lunch, which normally consisted of a bar of chocolate and a large hunk of cheese. On excluding these from her diet she immediately noticed a reduc- tion in frequency and severity of her migraine. She tried various other dietary exclusions and found that several foods seemed to be associated with her headaches. On avoiding fruit, alcohol and coffee in the week before her periods Lorna was delighted to find that her headaches were much less severe.

Migraine triggered by the chemicals in citrus fruit, cheese, chocolate, wheat, red wine and coffee is an established fact and is easy to prove by excluding them from the diet. Far more diffi- cult is trying to identify the whole host of other foods that trigger it. In Jackie's situation, removing these common foods from the diet did produce some reduction in attacks. This was not suffi- cient to completely relieve her suffering, but enough to suggest that food sensitivity could be the main trigger.

The first step was for Jackie to keep a diary of her headaches for a short time and to note down the food she had eaten in the previous 24 hours. It is important to record if there has been a particular craving for anything, as this may have been the food that causes the migraine attacks. It is straightforward dealing with people who can readily identify food triggers from a diary, as these are then avoided. In Jackie's case there was nothing particularly obvious, so it was necessary to try an exclusion diet.

This starts with a five-day period of virtual fasting which is designed to cleanse the system of any harmful food or chemicals that have been eaten. Ideally only spring water should be taken at this time, but complete lack of food often makes people feel ill so I allow them to eat pears and lamb. This is a strange combination, but neither of these have ever been shown to produce a food sensitivity. Foods are then reintroduced one at a time, with each meal consisting of one food only. You are then allowed to continue to eat any food that hasn't caused any immediate symptoms. There is enormous variation in the lists of foods that are incriminated in migraine and most people are allergic to more than one group of substances.

Jackie survived her five-day fast on pears and lamb, although she became fed-up with the sight of them. Her first meal was really cheating as she had chicken, carrots and potatoes but fortunately there was no reaction. At breakfast the following morning, a glass of grapefruit juice produced a mild headache which did not develop into a full-blow episode. Salad for lunch and ham for tea were fine but a piece of toast for the next breakfast produced a severe migraine which stayed with her all day. It was unfortunate that a bowl of cereal the next day produced another distressing attack. After a further few days of reintroducing her favourite foods it was clear that Jackie was sensitive to anything containing wheat or corn, and to a lesser extent to fruit. By excluding these totally from her diet she has remained free of headaches.

This technique will nearly always identify food sensitivity, and all migraine sufferers should try it at some stage. There are chemical tests that can be performed on the skin and blood to test for allergy, but these are expensive and not as reliable as the fasting method. Susceptibility can occur to any foodstuff but the commonest, apart from those described previously, are to nuts, wheat, corn, tomatoes, yeast, and milk and dairy produce.

By analysing and identifying the precipitating factors in migraine described above, it is quite possible to prevent the condition completely. Close attention must also be paid, as with all headaches, to the immune system which if in a depressed state will allow migraine to develop and prevent your own body defences from clearing it naturally. Steps to boost this are described in Chapters 3 and 4 and should be closely followed.

For Peter F., a 46-year-old central heating consultant, it was impossible to remove all the causes, especially as there was a great deal of tension and pressure at work. The business was struggling financially and it was highly stressful trying to keep it running in profit. He was unable to relax at home and his headaches occurred on most days. The medicines that Peter had taken in the past always made him feel dopey and unable to concentrate, so he wanted to know any non-drug therapy he could try. Here are some suggestions.

Visualization

As stress was the main cause of Peter's migraine, it was logical to try relaxation first. I have found, however, that the pain is usually too severe for simple relaxation to blot out. Visualization is a special form of relaxation using the formation of mental pictures to relieve the problem. A simple example is in athletes who improve their performance by seeing themselves at the Olympic Games winning the marathon to the roar of the huge crowd! When applied to migraine, this is extremely effective and first it is necessary to imagine the scene inside the brain that is producing the headaches. The pain is produced by constriction of the blood vessels, so one might visualize the enemy pushing on these arteries to narrow them. One lady I know then imagines her own cavalry, riding to her aid to repel the invaders. They are sent into retreat and the blood vessels can widen out again to normal. To be successful it is essential to visualize a positive outcome, as negative imaging can worsen the situation.

The other way to use visualization is to allow your mind to linger on a scene that is peaceful and tranquil. I always picture myself on a beach with the sun slowly rising above the horizon and the water gently lapping on the shore. For me the sun and the sea have been significant since my childhood and produce a feeling of calmness within, so in your own case pick out the elements that are meaningful to you.

Peter found that he could use both methods. At work, when his migraine started he would lean back in his chair and blow up the enemy forces with depth charges! At home, by picturing himself on the beach at Acapulco, he could achieve a very deep state of relaxation which relieved his headaches.

Self-hypnosis

This is the 'Rolls Royce' treatment for migraine and over the years I have found it to be the single most effective way of curing it. It is easy to learn, but until recently hypnosis has had a very bad image, mainly because of the highly inaccurate representation of it on television and films. People still believe that once in the hypnotic state, all control is lost and you are totally in the power of the therapist. This is completely untrue as you can never be made to do anything against your will or to say something too personal or private. Although some people are better hypnotic subjects than others, I have never found a patient who couldn't be hypnotized. Hypnosis is a level of consciousness somewhere between being awake and being asleep. It is a very relaxing experience, during which the therapist is able to communicate with your subconscious mind, and you can recall thoughts and events which otherwise would remain hidden. There are normally a number of barriers that prevent contact with the deeper parts of ourselves and it is these barriers that we can bypass using hypnosis.

Judith B. was a 45-year-old journalist, a career which she found stimulating and rewarding. Her husband worked as a director of an international engineering company, which involved both of them in a busy social life. This had increased dramatically in the previous six months with his promotion and Judith was finding it very difficult to combine her own job with running a home and frequent entertaining. Her migraine attacks had started many years previously but had never really caused serious problems until recently. When she came to the surgery her plight had become desperate as, every time they were due to go to an engagement, a severe headache would start and ruin the evening. Her husband was sympathetic at first but his patience soon wore thin as his partners became critical of his continual excuses. A number of different treatments had been prescribed including painkillers, antidepressants and tranquillizers with no improve-

ment, and there seemed little point in continuing to take medication if they were not helping her. Judith seemed an ideal
candidate to learn the technique of self-hypnosis, and I find that
it usually takes six sessions over a period of three weeks to achieve
a satisfactory hypnotic state which is deep enough to relieve the
headaches.

Like most people, Judith was convinced that it would be impossible for her to be hypnotized so I devoted the first appointment to convincing her that this was untrue. The first part of
hypnosis is known as induction and the most commonly used
method is to start with eye fixation. You focus on some object in
the room while the therapist talks gently and slowly and then after
a minute or two you will close your eyes and follow simple suggestions that are made. This usually involves simple exercises to slow
and regularize the breathing, and after a few minutes the hypnotic
state will be reached. Although this is not very deep to start with,
the depth will gradually increase as the treatment progresses. The
main advantage is that it is a very relaxed state in which it is easy
to respond to further suggestions that are made to you.

The remarkable thing about hypnosis and the main reason for
its success is that plans made during the session whilst in a
hypnotic state actually continue after the session is over. I stressed
to Judith again that I could not force her to do anything she didn't
want to and that she would feel in control of the situation at all
times. The skill in hypnosis is in taking the person back to different stages of their life to discover the reasons for the migraine. In
Judith's case, they had started at school with pressure around
exam time, and during the therapy I was able to free her of
negative thoughts and feelings about this time. Her headaches
had only flared again with the extra pressure on her at home
trying to impress her husband's business colleagues. I was able
to teach her positive thinking about this so that after the sessions
Judith would be left with the post-hypnotic suggestion that whenever the pressure started to build up she would automatically start
to relax.

After three-quarters of an hour I brought her out of hypnosis
and gradually back to normal consciousness. Judith was surprised that she had been under for so long, as it felt like only a
few minutes. I reassured her that she would not have any unpleasant effects from the experience and that only areas of life dealt

with during that treatment sessions would be affected by the hypnosis.

I could see that Judith was mystified by the thought of hypnotizing herself, but it is remarkable how quickly this technique can be learnt. It is really the key to success in the treatment of migraine. At her next appointment, her hypnotic state became considerably deeper now that most of her fears had been removed, and I was able to give her instructions that would enable her to hypnotize herself. These consisted of lying peacefully in a quiet room and taking a deep breath in and out followed by two normal ones. This cycle is repeated five times and by then she would be in a state of hypnosis. If anyone came into the room or disturbed her during this time then she would immediately become awake but some of the benefits would be lost. I advise a session of about fifteen minutes and strangely enough, you will automatically wake up after this length of time. In fact another patient of mine hypnotizes himself on the bus going to work in the morning and always wakes up just before his correct stop.

To relieve her headaches I set out the following plan for Judith. At the first sign of her migraine, or if in a situation where one always occurred, then she should immediately put herself into a state of self-hypnosis. This should be continued for ten minutes, then she would automatically return to normal consciousness, which I had previously taught her to do by slowly counting up to seven. This short time is often enough to clear the migraine but the effect can be reinforced in the hypnotic state by positively telling yourself that the headache will disappear. Suggestions like this introduced into the mind when it is clear of negative thoughts continue for hours or sometimes days after the hypnosis. As Judith became more practised she could quickly go into a very deep state of relaxation which immediately relieved her migraine, allowing her to go out and once again enjoy her demanding social life.

Many of my migraine sufferers have been treated successfully in this manner as self-hypnosis can be applied at any time, and indeed I often use it myself to relax between patients during a busy surgery.

Acupuncture

This is the best-known of all the alternative therapies and at long last is becoming accepted in the UK. It is extremely effective in controlling migraine, especially in people who feel averse to hypnosis. As acupuncture can also be used to treat other types of headache, I have described the theory in more detail in the chapter on special therapies and have restricted its application in this chapter solely to migraine.

John C. was a 40-year-old librarian who experienced severe one-sided headaches, mainly because of prolonged exposure to the stuffy atmosphere in the library. Like many sufferers, he had tried most of the available drugs without success and had read an article in his Sunday newspaper describing the beneficial effects of acupuncture. It had taken some time for him to come to the surgery as he wasn't keen on the idea of having several needles stuck into him! Acupuncture needles are in fact very thin and often no pain is felt when they pass through the skin. For John, I used five needles; three in the face and two in the right arm, which were left in for 20 minutes per session. I explained to John that if some part of him hurts then rubbing the affected part relieves the discomfort. Similarly with acupuncture, by gently stimulating the tender areas with the needles the pain is alleviated. This effect can last for several days after the treatment session and eventually, after several appointments, it will last for up to six months. All that is then needed is for a reinforcing dose of acupuncture to be given twice yearly.

Whilst some of the needles are put into the skin at the points of maximum intensity of the headaches, one or two are inserted at specific places in the body called acupuncture points. These have been plotted over many centuries by the Chinese and needling these will increase the effect many times over. By showing John the points that were specific to his own headaches, he was then able to use the technique of acupressure. This is basically massaging these points without the use of needles which, although not quite as effective, is still very useful. At any time, and especially at work, John had an active way of relieving his migraine. Rather than use simple finger massage, it is possible to use the blunt end of a matchstick for massage, taking care not to puncture the skin.

According to the theory of acupuncture, every part of the body is represented by a point in each ear and another useful trick in relieving headaches is to locate the part of the ear related to the head and to rub it quite hard. Some therapists will stick a stud into this point and leave it in situ by means of a small piece of sticking plaster. This can stay in place for about a fortnight and when the migraine starts the stud can be massaged in a circular manner. I remember at one dinner party a lady developing a severe migraine and she was absolutely amazed when it was relieved by simply rubbing vigorously on a part of her ear!

John improved tremendously following his course of acupuncture and it is now three months since his last significant headache. He has had a couple of minor attacks but these have been quickly relieved using acupressure. He has come to realize that his fears about the needles were groundless, but he did ask me once if they were adequately sterilized as he didn't want to catch anything from them. Fortunately, all acupuncture needles are now disposable and cannot be reused so there is no risk of cross-infection.

Homoeopathy

The range of patent medicines that are available for migraine is vast and most are worthless. Painkillers, tranquillizers, anti-emetics, antidepressants, and drugs to dilate the blood vessels in the brain have been produced, all of which have some damaging side-effects. In Western society we are brought up to believe the way to cure illness is to take a tablet, and it is difficult to convince people that there are other approaches. For this reason homoeopathy is very useful as, if used correctly, it is a fast and effective form of therapy. The theory of homoeopathy is explained in Chapter 11 on Special Therapies, but the real beauty of it is the lack of side-effects. It is difficult to buy the right sort of tablet for yourself without consulting a homoeopath first, as the choice depends only partly on the type of headache, and also on your personality and general lifestyle.

An example of this was Alison J. who was a 22-year-old student. Her symptoms were those of classical migraine with a hammering type of headache preceded or accompanied by flashing zigzags in front of the eyes and sometimes even a partial loss of vision. Her eyes tended to water and the symptoms were worse in the afternoon and evening. When asked about her health in general she revealed that she had rather greasy skin with a few spots and tended to be shy and nervous. The homoeopath usually looks for three features in a person and in Alison's case they were the classical migraine, the spotty skin and the nervous personality. On this basis she was prescribed Natrum Muriaticum and these, taken regularly, were very beneficial.

Debbie F. was also a student, but her migraine tended to start at the back of the head then spread over the top until it settled behind one eye. The headaches were associated with a bursting feeling and the whole head felt very sensitive. On general questioning Debbie said that her health was always worse in cold weather and she tended, usually, to feel chilly. Mental effort was difficult for her as she found it hard to concentrate and had a dread of failure. Her triad of symptoms therefore were a non-classical migraine, sensitivity to cold and a personality which lacked confidence. Silicea was the treatment of choice and proved extremely effective.

Anthony S. was a 53-year-old man who would wake up at weekends with an irritating migraine headache which, although not too severe, would be sufficient to stop enjoyment of his leisure time. His headache was always at the front of the head and felt rather constricting. It was usually accompanied by persistent nausea or vomiting and rather surprisingly was improved by moving about instead of more typically by rest. This 'Saturday morning' headache responds well to Iris Versicolor and Anthony was very pleased with its effect.

Monica C. had suffered from migraine before her periods since she was a teenager. These headaches were right-sided and started in the morning with some improvement through the day. The pain was improved by lying down or going to sleep. Monica described herself as very emotional and easily upset, and people of this type who experience premenstrual migraine benefit from Sanguinaria.

The main feature of Derek A.'s symptoms were that they became much worse on movement. Turning the head to one side led to a dramatic increase in the intensity of the pain, although pressure on the affected part of the head actually improved it. Derek had dark hair and a dark complexion and tended to be often thirsty with dry lips and a dry cough. He was perfect for the homoeopathic substance called Bryonia and the improvement on taking it was very dramatic.

I have described several examples of homoeopathic remedies to illustrate that there is a wide range available. People often complain that they don't work on them, but usually it is because they have taken one that is not suitable for their particular personality. If relief is not obtained quickly, it is well worth having one visit to a trained homoeopath who will be able to recommend the most suitable preparation. Further visits, which can prove very expensive, are not usually necessary.

Migraine is a horrible condition which destroys the quality of life. It is not easy to conquer, and finding a cure requires considerable time and effort. However, the methods for relief are not complicated and I have found without exception that everyone who is determined enough will master it so it no longer spoils their enjoyment of life.

Methods of relieving migraine

1) Eliminate precipitating factors:
   - the pill
   - excessive sleep
   - sunlight
   - alcohol
   - certain foods
   - seasonal variation
   - strenuous exertion
2) Visualization
3) Self-hypnosis
4) Acupuncture/acupressure
5) Homoeopathy

CHAPTER 8

Sinusitis

Whilst sinusitis cannot be classed as a serious medical condition, the constant aching headache and continually 'bunged up' feeling can make the sufferer feel extremely ill. It is socially unacceptable, as it sounds as though you have a heavy cold all the time and other people tend to keep their distance. The sinuses are responsible for the fluid or mucus that protects the lining of the nose. If this lining is attacked, which is usually by the common cold virus, then in response the body produces large quantities of mucus in an attempt to wash the viral particles away. Unfortunately the narrow passages leading from the sinus cavities to the nose are unable to cope with these extra secretions. They become blocked, leading to a build-up of mucus and the characteristic catarrh and associated severe headaches. Conventional drug therapy is aimed at drying up the mucus but all the medicines actually do is to thicken it which only makes the blockage worse with an increase in the intensity of the headaches.

A plan of action to clear the sinuses naturally is needed and this is well illustrated with the case of Geoff S. who is a 42-year-old teacher at a large primary school. Catching frequent colds is unfortunately an occupational hazard in this profession and Geoff was already on number five for this winter. With each one his sinuses were becoming more troublesome and when I saw him in the surgery he was unable to work as his frontal headaches had become so debilitating. The approach to this situation must be aimed at both preventing further attacks and removing the sinus blockage.

Geoff's lifestyle was by no means perfect, and this was certainly suppressing his immune system, leaving him wide open to recurrent infections. He found his job very stressful, but did little to try and relieve this pressure, and his diet was unplanned with a high proportion of 'junk food'. He took no regular exercise, as weekends were usually spent in bed trying to ward off his continual headaches. Subjected to this way of living, his body's defence system had little chance of fighting his sinus problem, and Geoff had therefore lost one of his major forces in his quest for improved health. To boost his immune system I advised him to follow the steps outlined in detail in chapters 2–5 consisting mainly of coping with stress, a wholefood diet, and regular exercise. For more specific treatment for sinusitis I advised Geoff on the various guidelines to follow.

Fresh air

Geoff liked walking in the country, although he never seemed to find enough free time. This is particularly beneficial for sinus headaches, as industrial pollutants like factory smoke and exhaust fumes inflame the linings of the nose which then become more susceptible to infection. The atmosphere in the country is much cleaner and Geoff found that if he spent part of his weekends in the hills, his head became clearer, and it was also beneficial to his high stress level. Cigarettes are a disaster for sinuses and the five a day that Geoff smoked were five too many.

Diet

A wholefood diet which is additive-free is essential, but there are some foods and drinks which increase the probability of sinus symptoms and these should be excluded. Dairy products, i.e. cow's milk and foods containing milk such as cheese, cream, butter and chocolate, together with sugar, sweets, artificial sweeteners, coffee and tea have all been implicated and should be avoided. When these products have built up for a considerable time, it is often necessary to have a short period of detoxification to cleanse the body. A 48-hour fast is quite adequate, taking in only fresh fruit juice and raw vegetables. This sounds drastic, but it enables the body to clear out all the toxic substances that have accumulated. The sinuses particularly become clogged up with poisonous germs, and these need to be removed before healing can take place.

For Geoff, who was a persistent sinus sufferer, his normal diet should include a large proportion of raw and fresh food. For example, breakfast should be a seed, nut and cereal mixture with fruit and a warm drink of herb tea. Main meals should include ample protein, preferably from a vegetable source such as pulses, although it can occasionally be from meat, poultry or fish. At least one of the main meals should include a large salad and desserts should usually be of fresh fruit. Occasionally everyone needs to go on a 'binge' and there is no real harm in this, but if this healthy diet is followed most of the time, then the sinuses will greatly benefit.

Supplements

Geoff had never taken any extra vitamins in his life, believing that his diet contained sufficient for his daily needs. Sinusitis sufferers have been shown to be deficient in vitamins A, B and C, so it is wise to boost the levels of these on a daily basis. Over the past few years I have recommended ginseng to patients. It has been used for generations in traditional Chinese medicine. One of the problems of sinusitis is that it can cause depression, and this can be counteracted by ginseng which is a natural though mild stimulant. It has an extra beneficial effect in regenerating the body's natural processes, and certainly most people feel better when taking it. Antibiotics tend to make the sinusitis worse and garlic, which is a natural antiseptic, is more effective. Four of the odour-free capsules should be taken daily.

Ionizers

Laura A. was a 20-year-old student who suffered with severe sinus headaches mainly above the eyes, radiating into the face. Every evening she had three to four hours' homework and found that this was becoming impossible as her concentration was seriously impaired by the pain. I advised her to purchase an ionizer and to keep this on continuously in her room. Ions are molecules that occur naturally in the air, some of which are positively charged and others negatively. Ionizers are small machines that produce a stream of negative ions and these reduce the levels of smoke, dust and harmful bacteria in the air by attaching themselves to these particles and rendering them harmless. This makes the air much purer and clearer to breathe. Recent surveys show that they cleared sinusitis in 60 per cent of sufferers and improved symptoms in over 80 per cent. In Laura's case this worked extremely well and at least there was one room in the house where she could gain relief. The main drawback to the use of ionizers is the limited area over which they are effective. It is not possible, obviously, to use them in every room, and they are ineffective outside.

Nasal washouts

If anyone ever asks me to suggest a single treatment which brings fast relief to sinus pain, I invariably advocate nasal douches. These are carried out by mixing a small amount of salt into a tumbler of tepid water. Sniffing the salt water up the nose makes it penetrate the sinus cavities, and when it is all blown back out again, the thick clogging mucus blocking the sinuses will be cleared and the headaches relieved. It is not a particularly pleasant procedure and is rather like inhaling sea water, but its effect is very dramatic and can work in a couple of minutes. Sometimes with longstanding sinusitis the lining of the nose becomes too tender to take salt water alone and a little beetroot juice can be added. If the soreness persists, then inhalation with a few drops of olbas oil in hot water is a suitable substitute for a short time to allow the delicate linings to recover. Nasal washouts should be performed daily until the symptoms are fully relieved.

Homoeopathy

Both Laura and Geoff needed some form of relief during the day and neither wanted to take conventional medicines because of troublesome side-effects. I remember myself once taking a decongestant tablet and spending several hours in a dry and sleepy state. The principle of homoeopathy is described in Chapter 11 but basically, as well as considering the main symptoms it also takes into account your personality and lifestyle. The tablets are free of any side-effects and can be taken safely. Laura's symptoms were worse in the evening and were improved by cold drinks and cold applications. She described herself as an emotional person easily moved to laughter or tears and admitted to being rather shy. These are the types of feature that the homoeopaths use for guidance and for this I prescribed Laura the preparation Pulsatilla which can be taken every half hour during an attack.

Geoff's symptoms typically started at the root of the nose and were associated with substantial sticky catarrh and severe nasal blockage. His headaches tended to be worse when he moved or stooped but were improved when he was out in the open air and ate hot food. He disliked the heat, had a yellowish tinge to his hair and was generally of a placid nature. This combination of features suggested that Kali Bichromicum would be the treatment of choice and this indeed proved effective.

Sinus headaches commonly occur in children and homoeopathic tablets can be used with the comforting knowledge that they will be free from damaging side-effects. An eight-year-old girl called Sarah came to the surgery with a combination of headaches across her forehead, burning eyes, and a nasal discharge of thick yellow mucus. Her mother commented that she was extremely restless and irritable which was different from her usual calm and precise nature. For this personality Silicea is beneficial and this proved to be the case for Sarah.

Homoeopathic preparations are many and varied so the reason for any lack of success in relieving headaches is invariably because an unsuitable one has been prescribed. It is well worth analysing your personality and picking out the relevant features. Then, by looking in your local library at a homoeopathic reference book, you can find the right preparation for you. They are inexpensive and easily obtained from any health food shops and some chemists.

Acupressure

My first introduction to complementary medicine was when I learned acupuncture and over the years I have tried to develop a method of teaching patients a technique known as acupressure. This is carried out by massaging a series of acupuncture points without actually inserting any needles. It is gentle, painless and invariably very relaxing. Laura was a suitable person to benefit as she often found that her sinus headaches would come on very quickly at times of high stress during the day.

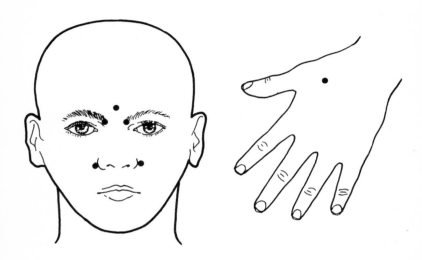

Acupuncture points

First I proved to Laura that acupuncture is effective by seeing her at a time when her headache was at its worst and relieving it with three needles in her face and one in her left hand. At the next appointment Laura used the tip of a finger instead of the needles and applied firm pressure in an upward or circular motion to the same points. This pressure should be applied to each place for half to one minute before moving to the next point, so the whole treatment only takes two or three minutes. The exact sites for the massage are easy to find as they are tender to press. The first location is in the middle of the forehead about one centimetre above the top of the nose, the second at the inner corner of the eyebrow, and the third is at the base of the nose. As is common in acupuncture, a distant point is used and for sinus headaches it is at the base of the thumb. These are clearly shown in the diagram. Laura was able to use this technique several times a day whenever her headaches started and wherever she was working. Occasionally this method of stimulation is not sufficient, and a full course of acupuncture is required. However, this is not usually necessary and for Laura regular acupressure produced tremendous relief despite her initial scepticism.

Conventional medicine has completely failed to cope with the problem of sinusitis and the accompanying headaches. When conventional drug therapy fails, usually the specialist turns to surgery, which means widening out the narrow channels that carry the mucus from the sinus cavities to the nose. This is unpleasant, requiring a few days' stay in hospital, and in my opinion is not necessary. I only mention this here as patients come into see me in great fear of having any surgery performed on them. The one thing that can be beneficial is a simple sinus washout which completely clears the sinus cavities and allows healing to take place. Appropriate steps can then be taken to prevent the mucus building up again. Horror stories abound about washouts, but they are quick and painless. Cotton wool soaked in local anaesthetic, usually cocaine, is pushed up each nostril and after a few minutes a small tube is passed into each sinus down which a salt solution is squirted under pressure flushing out the mucus. The whole process only takes five minutes and the only after-effect is slight dizziness.

Sinusitis responds to the self-help methods described above and only rarely is it necessary to seek expert assistance. The main message is that it can be effectively treated, and the nagging headaches that stop you living life to the full can be abolished.

Methods of relieving sinusitis

1) Fresh air
2) Diet — avoid dairy produce
3) Supplements
4) Ionizers
5) Nasal washouts
6) Homoeopathy
7) Acupressure

CHAPTER 9

High blood pressure

High blood pressure, if ignored, can be a killer: it may cause a stroke or heart attack. In most people who suffer from this condition, the level is only raised by a small amount and it will revert to normal by using various natural methods. The section on high blood pressure in Chapter 1 of this book briefly described some of the self-help techniques available, and in this section I would like to look at these in more detail with special reference to a 48-year-old patient of mine.

Penny T. was a social worker who was keen on sport and found that it was an excellent method of unwinding after the stresses of her job. Twelve months previously she had developed severe generalized headaches which made her feel as if her head was going to explode. They were present on waking, lasted throughout the day and sometimes made her dizzy. These headaches were most suggestive of raised blood pressure and this was confirmed when measurement showed it to be 200/105. Penny asked me to explain these figures to her as she had no idea of the normal level.

Blood pressure is a reflection of how hard the heart has to work to pump blood around the body and is measured with an instrument called a sphygmomanometer. A cuff is wrapped around the upper arm and inflated until it completely compresses all the blood vessels, acting in the same way as a tourniquet. The cuff is slowly released and, as the pressure reduces the blood vessels start to open. This makes a characteristic sound which can be heard at the elbow, and when all the vessels have opened, the sound ceases. The level at the onset of the sound is the top level — in Penny's case it was 200 — and the level at the disappearance of the sound is the bottom figure, which was 105. If the arteries are narrowed or thickened, they take greater pressure to constrict them and the measurements rise. This usually occurs either from a furring up of the channels or, more commonly, by spasm of the muscles in the blood vessel walls. A normal blood pressure for Penny should not exceed 140/90 although it does not become dangerous until it rises above 170/100. Conventional medicine cannot explain the reason for a rise in blood pressure, but as the artery walls are encircled by muscle it would seem that anything that causes these to tighten will increase blood pressure, and conversely, when this muscle is relaxed, the blood pressure level will fall.

Penny's doctor had treated her with tablets, with an excellent reduction in pressure, but they had made her feel tired and lethargic. This was tolerable at work but the enjoyment of her sporting activities was spoiled to a degree where it was difficult to carry on playing. A change in the type of drug taken had not improved the situation, and anyway, she did not like the idea of taking medicine for the rest of her life. Penny asked me if there was a natural way of dealing with high blood pressure and I formulated a simple and practical plan for her.

All the steps described in Chapters 2–5 should be taken to boost the immune system, i.e. a wholefood diet, regular exercise, and stress reduction. With each of these, however, there are special recommendations for high blood pressure, and these are detailed below.

Nutrition

A healthy diet is a major key to reducing the level of pressure, and there are several foodstuffs that are undesirable. These include refined products, like white flour or sugar, and all types of fats. Eating these has been shown to produce damage to blood vessel walls as well as resulting in obesity, both of which are major factors in the development of high blood pressure. An excessive intake of red meat sends the level up, and a recent survey showed that vegetarians have a significantly lower blood pressure than meat eaters. A vegetarian diet contains a much higher intake of potassium, which is significant in maintaining a reduction of pressure in these individuals. The intake of alcohol should not exceed two units per day.

I advised Penny that this left a diet in which the helpful foods include: the low-fat proteins, such as fish, chicken, and low-fat cheeses; all vegetables and fruits; and the whole range of grains, seeds, nuts and pulses. For many people this means a major change in dietary pattern, and should be adopted over a period of several weeks.

Salt

I have separated this from general nutrition as it is so important. Penny was a great lover of liberally sprinkling salt on her food at the table, thereby greatly increasing her intake of sodium. This tends to hold fluid in the body and increases the amount of blood in the arteries, producing a rise in blood pressure. It is unlikely that a very small amount of salt added to cooking will be detrimental but it must be banished from the table!

Supplements

Certain of these have a lowering effect on pressure and also aid the functioning of the heart. Vitamin C in the dose of 1g daily, vitamin E: 200 micrograms (μg) daily and vitamin B complex: 1 tablet daily or brewer's yeast: 8 tablets per day should all be taken regularly. As Penny was not a vegetarian, I also advised vitamin B_{13} which contains extra potassium, and two garlic capsules each morning.

Smoking

Unfortunately, one of the methods Penny used to relax after a hard day at work was to light a cigarette. Smoking has a direct and dramatic effect on blood pressure, and the level can rise by 25 points within seconds of the first puff. Nicotine produces an increase in adrenaline which has a constricting action on arteries. Heavy smokers will notice that their hands and feet are continually cold as a consequence. Even worse is that repeated smoking will eventually lead to a raised level of adrenaline in the body which does not fall at the end of the cigarette.

Exercise

Physical exertion is beneficial as it boosts the immune system, but certain forms of exercise will also lower the blood pressure. Walking on a regular basis can lower the level by 20 points even if it only involves a trip to the local shops. Everyone who can walk should do so whenever possible and at least 30 minutes every other day is ideal. The long-term blood pressure response to such activity is to stay reduced as a result of an increased efficiency of the circulatory system and a relaxation of the muscles in the artery walls. Penny liked walking but rarely found the time so I urged her to walk the mile and a half to work each day. Her main sport was badminton and this was fine, although a word of warning to her was never to play squash, as the sudden severe exertion can lead to a major rise in blood pressure. Cycling and swimming are alternatives, although neither have been shown to be as effective as walking.

Rest and relaxation

Stress is without doubt the single most significant factor in raising blood pressure. The simplest way of reducing this is to ensure that you have adequate rest and sleep. Penny usually went to bed late and was only averaging five hours' sleep per night. Depending on individual needs the amount of sleep required varies, but in a demanding lifestyle should be between six and eight hours daily. People who live in countries where a siesta is usually taken have a great advantage, as a rest in the middle of the day can drop the mean blood pressure reading. Obviously in Britain a siesta is not possible for most people, but a basic relaxation exercise can be used during the lunch break with an equally beneficial effect. Penny tended to work through her lunch hour in an effort to keep up with her work and also was having problems falling asleep, so her resting time was considerably shorter than was needed. At the surgery I keep a stock of cassette tapes describing various relaxation techniques and I lent one to Penny which was equally suitable for use at work and at home. These cassettes last only about ten minutes and produce a feeling of inner calm. Penny found that she rarely reached the end of the tape at night before falling asleep.

I have described in detail the various relaxation techniques in Chapter 6, but a cassette recording is a short cut. These are cheap to buy and can be obtained from most health food shops. When she used these various steps to lower her blood pressure, Penny's level fell inside three months to 135/85 which was within normal levels. This then removed the risk of a stroke or heart attack, but I stressed to her the importance of keeping this routine going or her blood pressure would rise again. With the reduction to normal her headaches completely disappeared, and consequently the quality of her life was greatly improved.

Sometimes these simple methods do not lower the blood pressure sufficiently, and more advanced techniques are necessary. Nick V. was aged 41 when he came into the surgery with severe headaches and a blood pressure of 215/110. I went through the same routine as with Penny but his pressure only reduced to 165/100. This was a considerable improvement, but was not yet below the upper limits of 140/90.

Autogenic exercises

This is a much stronger form of relaxation that is not necessary purely for the relief of stress, but it has been shown to reduce significantly stubborn cases of high blood pressure. A reclining position should be adopted with the eyes closed, and distracting external sounds should be minimized. The exercises involve the use of specific verbalized messages to focus awareness on a particular area. No effort is involved, but simply a passive concentration on any sensations or emotions that may result from each message. This may sound complicated but in practice is relatively straightforward. When a sequence of autogenic or self-generated instructions are combined with the passive aspect of meditation, a powerful method of blood pressure reduction is created.

The process starts with a general thought such as 'I feel relaxed and peaceful' and this is followed by concentrating on a specific area of the body such as the arm. Repeat to yourself several times that the arm feels warm. To encourage this feeling of warmth it is useful to imagine the sun's rays shining on the back of the hand warming it. Proceed through the whole body, pausing for some seconds at each area to experience the sensation of increasing heat. When a part of the body becomes warm, the peripheral blood flow is increased and the muscles around the arteries relax. This produces a quite significant fall in blood pressure.

Whilst he was learning this approach I reassured Nick that certain areas of the body would be more responsive than others and that it would take several weeks to fully learn the technique. Persistence, patience and a total lack of urgency are all that is required to lead to a decrease in blood pressure and the relief of headaches.

Homoeopathy

Nick had always believed that illness was easily cured by taking tablets, and this is still the attitude of most of the populace. Homoeopathic preparations have the advantage of satisfying this need without the danger of side-effects. I have described the theory in Chapter 11 on Special Therapies, but Nick was a clear-cut example of how this theory can be applied in practice. He was a lively, entertaining person most of the time, but when his head-aches developed Nick became bad-tempered and even violent. In fact, whenever he felt ill from any cause he became red-faced and his whole head felt hot and painful. At the same time, his mouth would go dry and there would be an associated hacking cough. The headaches were always worse on waking and were aggravated by noise, touch and motion. Here, therefore, was the triad of symptoms that every homoeopath looks for; the particular features of the headache, physical appearance, and personality. Only then can the person be treated as a whole and the correct medication chosen. In this instance Belladonna was the treat-ment of choice and would have been the only homoeopathic remedy of much value.

In general I am not particularly happy about patients selecting their own preparations and treating themselves when high blood pressure is involved. It is difficult to identify the characteristics of your own personality that are relevant and the failure of the tablets is often because the wrong choice has been made. A single appointment with a homoeopath is well worth while as this will identify the important facets of your condition so you know that the correct preparation is being taken. As homoeopaths are nearly always private it is not really advisable to keep going for repeated visits as a large bill can soon be accumulated.

Nick was happy with the Belladonna and, over the following three months, by taking these during the day and practising the autogenic exercises early evening, he brought his blood pressure down to within normal limits.

Acupuncture

Jack E. was a 53-year-old man who came for treatment of his headaches by a course of acupuncture. His blood pressure was 190/110 and he had no desire to take any medication. He had lived in China for over twenty years so was convinced that acupuncture was the treatment of choice in his case. I was apprehensive about using this method for high blood pressure, but my tutor always claimed that needling in the correct places would bring a rapid and sustained fall in pressure. Four points were used — one in the centre of the forehead, one behind the ear, the third at the back of the neck and the last on the forearm just above the wrist. The needles were stimulated using a low electric current for twenty minutes at a time, and it required three treatments before any improvement was noticed in the blood pressure readings. Jack was a man of great faith and never doubted that the acupuncture would be successful. At the end of the sixth appointment his pressure was down to 145/80 and I have been able to maintain this by giving him a treatment session once a month.

These same four points could be massaged at home without the use of needles — a technique called acupressure. This involves rubbing the acupuncture point with the tip of the finger for one to two minutes at a time and then moving on to the next one. Jack, like an increasing number of people, had bought his own machine for measuring blood pressure. These are relatively inexpensive and in this age of electronics all that is required is to inflate a cuff on the arm and release the pressure. The blood pressure readings are then shown automatically on the dial. This is an excellent way of showing response to treatment, as whenever patients come to the surgery for a check there is always some degree of tension which automatically tends to increase the blood pressure. This gives a falsely high reading and a mistaken impression that the treatment is insufficient.

In my experience, following the plan outlined in the two cases above will nearly always lower blood pressure sufficiently to remove any need for drug therapy. The associated headaches will be automatically relieved as the pressure falls. Once again it is an illustration that headaches are not a disease in themselves, but are a sign that all is not well in the body. On many occasions I have seen patients in the surgery who have taken painkillers over a period of years to try to cure their headaches without once looking for the underlying cause. Any headache which is 'bursting' in nature and associated with dizziness warrants a blood pressure check. Just occasionally the level can be so high that there is immediate danger and drugs may have to be used in the short term. However, by using the different self-help techniques described, the use of patent medicines need only be temporary and long-term side-effects can be avoided. To lower blood pressure to a normal level takes considerable time and effort, but it is a potentially serious condition, so the time and effort is worth it. To be able to manage it naturally, by leading a healthier lifestyle, is an added bonus.

Methods of controlling high blood pressure

1) Nutrition
2) Low salt intake
3) Dietary supplements
4) No smoking
5) Regular exercise
6) Rest and relaxation
7) Autogenic exercises
8) Homoeopathy
9) Acupuncture

CHAPTER 10

Other headaches

The fact that other causes of headaches are less common does not make them any less significant or unpleasant. Some can be managed using natural therapies, although occasionally it is necessary to turn to conventional methods. Where appropriate I have indicated the situations where this is advisable and what the likely outcome will be.

Cervical spondylosis

The head is able to turn by using the muscles in the neck. Obviously, if the neck were a single straight bone, movements would be extremely limited, so to enable it to bend it is made up of a number of bones called vertebrae with a 'rubber' pad in between them. The muscles in the scalp originate from these vertebrae, so if anything goes awry in the neck then spasm is produced in these muscles and a severe headache develops.

Posture

Alice F. was a 56-year-old woman who had worked as a clerical officer for the local council for over twenty years. This involved spending all day at a desk sorting through papers and files. Over the previous two years she had noticed a gradually worsening pain in her neck with an accompanying severe headache spreading over the top of her scalp. This increased in intensity as the day wore on. I explained to Alice that the development of this situation is invariably related to a defect in posture, and in her case it was from sitting in a poorly-constructed chair, making her hunch over her desk. This was first recognized earlier this century by a man called Alexander who suggested that a great deal of modern illness can be traced to the posture of the body. Muscles are tense when they should not be, vertebrae are contracted together, the neck is sunk into the chest and legs are constantly crossed and turned in. Whilst it is hard to accept that this is the root of all illness, it is certainly the main precipitating factor in cervical spondylosis. I explained to Alice how she should try and correct her neck problem so as to relieve her headaches.

Everyone knows that we should stand up straight without hunching, but the problems really start when we sit down. Most chairs are designed for one reason only, and that is to increase sales. Furthermore, most people buy furniture because of its appearance, and when no one is sitting in it! By the age of 11 years, over 70 per cent of children show marked muscular and postural difficulties. Take a look at anyone sitting down and you will see any of the following: a rounded back, compressed stomach, and the thighs at an angle of less than 90 degrees to the trunk. I stressed to Alice that the crux of having a good posture lay in opening out this angle. An angle of 135 degress is ideal: it frees the spine and allows the neck to have a full and unrestricted range of movement. Children often do this automatically, by tilting ordinary four-legged chairs so they are sitting over the front legs with the back ones in the air, in an attempt to bring the body into a more natural position. Back support is unnecessary when the thigh/trunk angle is in balance, since the freed spine lengthens and finds its own natural position. I urged Alice to buy a Balans chair for work, which is a chair with a tilted seat, a rest for the lower legs and no back. This automatically produces the correct angle between legs and trunk, thus freeing the neck and preventing that terrible hunching over the desk. These chairs have the great advantage of being much cheaper than conventional ones. She was amazed to find that, after two weeks, her headaches had virtually disappeared.

Physiotherapy

Attention to posture is often all that is required, but after many years, arthritis of the neck may develop, which will require more intensive treatment. This happened to a 68-year-old patient of mine called Catherine W., and I initially prescribed a course of physiotherapy using deep heat which produced a relaxation of the muscles and a reduction in inflammation. There are several types of machine, and at my own practice we use either a short wave or interferential. The standard infra-red lamps that many people have at home are effective in relaxing the muscles, but are very limited in their depth of penetration and are therefore not as beneficial. Many surgeries now employ their own physiotherapist so that this treatment can be obtained quickly when required.

Osteopathy

Catherine responded quite well to physiotherapy, but one of the complications of spinal conditions is that nerves can be trapped between the small joints. This is the reason why tablets and simple remedies are ineffective. To relieve this I considered referring Catherine to an osteopath whose speciality is to deal with problems associated with bones, joints and ligaments by manipulation. This is really a form of bloodless surgery which frees the joints and allows the trapped nerve to be freed. The only drawback to osteopathy is that a reasonable amount of force has to be used, which can produce discomfort for a few days after therapy. This may be necessary for rugby players, but for some-one of Catherine's disposition I preferred the gentler technique of a chiropractor.

Chiropractic

This works on the principle of seeking out misalignments in the bones of the neck and correcting them. When a joint is found to be slightly out of place it can be restored to normal by an ex-tremely light yet rapid springing motion known as the toggle recoil. The pressure is not more than a light nudge and often the patient may wonder if anything has been done at all. The effect is often dramatic and there are no unpleasant after-effects. Catherine needed only three visits before her headaches disappeared and now goes only occasionally if the pain recurs. For the particularly resistant patient, the chiropractor uses a special technique called cranial osteopathy which is a very gentle method of working on the different bones of the skull. It involves cradling the head and very subtly making miniscule adjustments to glide the bones of the skull into the correct position. This will enable the neck to relax and resume its normal posture which brings complete relief of the headaches.

Acupuncture

Cervical spondylosis is a condition which responds especially well to acupuncture. The neck is the place in the body where several of the acupuncture channels come together so the needles have an extremely strong and lasting effect. It is only necessary to use four needles, one each on either side of the back of the neck, one in the middle of the neck and the fourth at the base of the thumb on the side where the pain is worse. Stimulation is gentle for about fifteen minutes and normally about four treatments are necessary.

Methods of controlling cervical spondylosis

1) Good posture
2) Physiotherapy
3) Osteopathy
4) Chiropractic
5) Acupuncture

Eye problems

Eye-strain is a frequent cause of headaches, especially in teenagers. Andy F. was 14 years old when first seen, and the fact that the headaches had built up gradually over a period of months had led the parents to fear a brain tumour, but the pain was situated above and around the eyes which is not typical of a lesion inside the skull. Surprisingly, although it is often the case, Andy denied any visual problems but on testing was found to be short-sighted.

The logical treatment is to prescribe glasses, but this can often be avoided by ensuring that the body is kept in good condition. The eyes generally reflect the person's vitality, and eye problems can indicate an unhealthy lifestyle with subsequent suppression of the immune system. I stressed to Andy the importance of following the steps outlined in Chapters 2-5 which basically include a wholefood diet, regular exercise and a more relaxed lifestyle. The eye muscles tire very easily, and adequate rest is essential. Most teenagers like to go to parties, but it is vital to have sufficient sleep on the other nights. Fortunately Andy followed these recommendations and his eye-strain settled.

In older patients, headaches are often caused by a build-up of pressure in the eyes — a condition called glaucoma. Ethel P. developed this at the age of 76 and I explained to her that this was a serious condition. It was imperative for her to go to a specialist or optician to have the pressures checked as, if glaucoma is not treated, blindness can ultimately ensue. Ethel did not want to take drugs at her age, but although there is no naturally safe way of relieving the pressure, all that is needed is an instillation of special eye drops once or twice daily to keep the level normal. At least this is a 'cure' without the risk of side-effects. Happily Ethel's eyes have returned to normal pressure and her headaches have disappeared.

Infection

Any acute infection can cause headaches, however minor, so it is nothing to become too concerned about. It does seem, however, that if the immune system is not functioning to full capacity, the headaches develop much more easily, and this is yet another reason why we owe it to ourselves to keep it in tip-top shape.

Teeth

A number of research projects have suggested, though it has not been proven, that many headaches are caused by problems with the teeth. Dental problems can lead to abnormalities in the function of the joint between the jaw and the skull. This is a simple hinge joint which undergoes an enormous amount of stress during a lifetime and if it opens incorrectly it will produce both muscular and migraine-type headaches. As a result, many patients have been treated with specially-designed plates to try to correct the way the jaw moves. It is difficult to assess their effectiveness and this technique must remain unproven. The best advice is that if your headaches do not fall into an obvious category, then it is well worth having your teeth checked. Only contemplate this form of treatment if your dentist recommends it, and only if you trust him or her!

Trauma

It may seem obvious that a blow to the head will produce a headache and this is usually transient, caused by bruising of the scalp muscles. If the trauma is more severe it may cause concussion, where the brain itself is shaken up. Kevin Z. was a goalkeeper in a local football team and was knocked unconscious by the boot of an opposing forward one Saturday afternoon. He made a quick recovery and was able to play again the following weekend. Six months later he came to the surgery complaining of persistent generalized headaches which seemed to have started soon after the injury. He did not realize that post-concussion headaches can last for months and occasionally years. The brain is a very sensitive organ and does not like being kicked! I gave Kevin a course of acupuncture using six needles strategically placed on the scalp, and this considerably relieved his pain.

Temporal arteritis

I make no apology for mentioning this condition again as it has such potentially serious complications. Minnie D. was a 74-year-old whom I saw on a visit one Saturday. She was complaining of a severe throbbing headache over the left temple and had been sick several times. Minnie had a long history of migraine and it seemed reasonable to assume that this was another attack. I was suspicious, however, as the headache was higher up the forehead than usual and her usual migraine tablets had been ineffective. I went back to see her the following day by which time she had developed tender thickening of the temporal artery which could be felt throbbing in her left temple. This particular blood vessel supplies the eye and when it becomes inflamed it can sometimes block completely, thus removing the blood supply to the eye on that side. This results in sudden blindness. The only effective treatment is to use high doses of cortisone, and this should always be started if there is any suspicion of this condition. Fortunately Minnie settled quickly after the treatment commenced and she did not develop any eye problems. I have seen two blind people who weren't so lucky and it is a tragedy when this occurs because the steroids were not given early enough.

Sub-arachnoid haemorrhage

This is a condition which is caused by a congenital weakness in a blood vessel in the brain, which typically bursts between the ages of 30 and 40. The classical symptom is the sensation that someone has punched you on the back of the neck, and this is followed by increasing neck stiffness. This is a potentially fatal condition as further bleeding may arise, leading to brain damage. If there is suspicion of this then hospital admission is needed urgently for investigation. If this weakness is found, then the only course is an operation to repair it. Although this sounds catastrophic, in actual fact it is a very safe surgical procedure with a full recovery.

Brain tumours

Again I have left these to last as they are so uncommon. Alex C. was 18 when he presented with severe generalized headaches, vomiting and weight loss. Examination revealed signs of increased pressure inside the skull and investigations at the hospital revealed a cancerous tumour in the frontal region of the brain. His parents immediately expected the worst but were amazed when the specialist explained that this tumour could be removed. Alex had his operation the following day and made a full recovery. That was nine years ago, and he has not been troubled since. I would not pretend that all brain tumours are curable but certainly many are, either with surgery or radiotherapy, so one must never look at the situation with anything but an optimistic attitude. Furthermore, many of them turn out not to be cancerous which means they will not spread, and their removal is easier for the surgeon.

Headaches usually have a simple and non-serious cause, but even when there is a potentially dangerous situation, as long as they are approached speedily and logically, it is possible to cure all but a tiny number.

CHAPTER 11

Special therapies

In the preceding chapters I have recommended different types of alternative therapies that are effective in relieving headaches. These avoid the use of potentially toxic drugs, which merely suppress the symptoms rather than treating the cause of the illness. As we are human beings and not machines there is always some individual variation to the different treatments. It is for this reason that I have described more than one type for each condition and it is often a case of personal preference as to which you try first. Some people are convinced that acupuncture will work for them whereas others will be frightened by the needles so might try homoeopathy instead.

The number of alternative therapies available can cause problems to the prospective patient, and it is easier to choose if you have a basic knowledge of the theory of each one. Unfortunately, as the law in Britain stands at present, anyone can call themselves an acupuncturist or osteopath etc., without any training or qualifications, and set up in practice. Before starting the treatment don't be afraid to ask how long the person has been in practice and what sort of problems they are used to dealing with.

This chapter explains the principles of each kind of therapy and it also lists some organizations. I would strongly recommend writing to these for a list of qualified practitioners in your own area as this only takes a few days and will guarantee you a certain standard of treatment. One of the major reasons for the failure of a particular therapy is because it has been poorly administered, and someone can be put off for life by a treatment that could really be very beneficial. Most practitioners have the patients' interests at heart but regrettably, as in any walk of life, a few are only in it for a quick profit. In Britain, there is very little alternative medicine available on the NHS so it is easy to run up a large bill if you keep returning for more sessions. This is all right if you are improving, but some practitioners will try to convince you that you need to come back time and again until your money runs out. As a general guide I feel that a marked benefit should have been felt within four appointments, and if this is not the case then that particular therapy should be abandoned. I am not necessarily saying that your headaches will be cured, but they should be diminishing both in intensity and frequency.

Acupuncture

This is the best-known of all the alternative therapies and has been in use in China for thousands of years. In the West it is practised by three groups: medical doctors who have studied it at postgraduate courses, physiotherapists, and lay acupuncturists. The training of the last group varies enormously, from those who have undertaken full training lasting several years to those who have only taken a correspondence course. In theory it is better to go to qualified doctors as they have gone through exhaustive training at medical school and at least they will know what they are sticking the needles into! However, it does not necessarily mean that someone without a qualification is incompetent as I have known some brilliant natural healers. Listed in this chapter are the main organizations that will supply you with a registered list of practitioners.

Acupuncture is totally different from Western medicine. We are conventionally taught that our bodies are made up of various organs that derive their nutrients and therefore energy from the blood that passes through them. In contrast, Chinese medicine maintains that the health of any living thing depends on the flow of a life force or energy around the body. This energy is called 'Qi' (which is pronounced *chee*) and is passed to different organs via a series of channels rather like a railway system. Each of these channels starts in the hand or foot and follows a different route to eventually finish in the brain. If illness or injury occurs then there will be an interruption of flow of Qi in that particular channel.

The aim of acupuncture is to restore this flow of energy and then normal health will resume. At various points along its route, every channel comes close to the surface of the body and it is at these points that needles can be passed into them. When the point enters the channel the patient experiences a change of sensation, either a numbness or tingling, and this is termed 'needling sensation'. If the needle is stimulated either by gently twisting it or by using an electric current, energy can be produced thus restoring normal balance and allowing the body to heal itself.

Taking a headache above the left eye as an example, this indicates that there is an obstruction to the flow of Qi in the channel that passes through this area. This particular one is called the heart channel and starts in the hand. To relieve the obstruction, it is usual to insert about four needles — three around the painful area in the face, and the fourth at the nearest point to the beginning of the channel in the hand. The needles are very fine and can hardly be felt passing through the skin. These are stimulated intermittently for about twenty minutes and are then removed. All acupuncture needles are now disposable and are discarded after each treatment, so there is no chance of cross-infection. Some improvement is often felt after the first treatment and a course is usually of 4–6 treatments.

It is interesting that many of the main acupuncture points become tender when disease affects part of the body. It is quite possible to massage these points with the finger rather than using needles and I often teach my patients to do this. It is is not as effective or as long-lasting as needles but it does nevertheless produce marked benefit and can be carried out at any time.

All the acupuncture channels have a surface point in the ear and it is possible to restore the imbalance of energy by stimulating a single needle placed in the appropriate point. This is located by the use of a blunt probe which is pressed on to the skin of the ear until an acutely painful point is found. This will be the point of entry into the correct channel.

I well remember being at a dinner party and becoming thoroughly irritated by one lady constantly complaining of her toothache. I used the blunt end of a matchstick to locate the sensitive spot in her ear, and a firm massage completely cleared the pain.

Chinese medicine varies in other ways in that whereas we might think in terms of a virus invading the body, the Chinese describe the illness as various types of weather. Do not be surprised, when you go for your consultation, if the acupuncturist decides that your muscular headache is due to an invasion by wind. Alternatively, if the ache is caused by an infection, it is a disease of heat. Before there is any use of needles, the therapist will endeavour to establish the nature of the energy imbalance. Particular attention will be paid to the pulse and the tongue and these are looked at in quite a different way from the way your own doctor looks at them. Pulse diagnosis is performed at the wrist, and according to the Chinese you have a total of twelve different pulses. There are three superficial and three deep pulses to each arm and one of these relates to one of the organs or systems of the body. As described above, each organ also relates to a channel so there are always three things to be considered together: organ, channel and pulse. By recognizing abnormalities in the pulses, the acupuncturist can identify the organ and channel that is affected. The colour and character of the tongue are also valuable diagnostic pointers in assessing energy imbalance.

Sometimes if you are suffering from a disease of cold, as in migraine, it is necessary to introduce heat into the channel to correct this effect. This can be done by heating the needles using a substance called moxa or occasionally by placing it directly on to the skin. so you can appreciate that it is not simply a question of sticking a few needles in at random, and for this reason it is vital to consult a well trained and qualified therapist. I have listed the organizations to write to below for a register of practitioners.

The British Acupuncture Association
34 Alderney Street, London SW1V 4EU

Register of Traditional Chinese Medicine
74 Thorndean Street, London SW18 4HE

Traditional Acupuncture Foundation
American City Building, Columbia MD21044, USA

Australian Traditional Medicine Society
Rozelle, Victoria

Homoeopathy

All over the world the use of homoeopathic medicine is growing rapidly and is practised both by doctors and lay practitioners. In

Britain, homoeopathic treatment has been available under the NHS for many years and the preparations are available on prescription. Although only a few general practitioners practise it in their surgeries, this number is increasing all the time. In addition there are many private therapists so it should be easy to find one in your own area.

Homoeopathic treatment is based on the 'like cures like' principle where an illness or disease is treated with a remedy which may itself cause similar symptoms. This may sound nonsensical at first but it is really quite straightforward and is based on similar principles to vaccinations. If your children are vaccinated against measles, they are actually injected with a very small dose of the measles virus. This is not severe enough to cause an actual attack of the disease, but is sufficient to stimulate a particular response in the body's immune system. If the body is ever challenged again by the virus it already has a mechanism in place ready to fight it off. Homoeopathy works in the same way, where you take in a very low strength of a substance and the body reacts to fight off any diseases which have the same symptoms.

Other factors have to be taken into consideration and the homoeopath will go into the details of the complaint rather more comprehensively than other practitioners would. Details of your personality and general lifestyle will be considered; for example whether you are shy and nervous or more self-confident, whether you are sensitive to heat or cold and if you prefer the outdoors. From all this information the therapist will build up a total picture of you and only then will be able to decide the appropriate remedy.

Most homoeopathic tablets are taken every day for a period of time or in some cases continually to reinforce the effect on the body's immune system. Occasionally, if the preparation is very potent, it may only be prescribed in the dose of one tablet a month, and people become dismayed as they think they are not having sufficient. It is unusual to have to take more than one type of tablet at a time and I am always very suspicious of practitioners who prescribe combination therapy. These therapists also tend to give the preparations numbers and not names so you can only go back to them for further supplies. Homoeopathic tablets are of very low strength as only a microscopic amount of the substance is required to stimulate the protective reaction. For this reason they are very safe and completely free from side-effects. They have the added advantage of being cheap to buy.

Throughout this book I have described the particular remedy to take for each condition but it is important to learn how to take them. The tablet is placed in the mouth and allowed to dissolve slowly. On no account should it be swallowed, as it will be destroyed by the acid in the stomach. During a headache the medication should be taken every two hours, and for more chronic conditions three times daily is adequate. Toothpaste and cigarettes should be avoided for at least an hour before the tablets and under no circumstances should they be handled, but tipped into the lid of the container and dropped into the mouth.

If you decide to treat yourself without consulting a practitioner it is important to realize that the reason the treatment may fail is because the incorrect preparation has been chosen, and not because homoeopathy is unsuitable for your problem.

Addresses to write to for practitioners in your area are:

The British Homoeopathic Association
27a Devonshire Street, London W1N 1RJ

The Hahnemann Society
Humane Education Centre, Avenue Lodge,
Bounds Green Road, London W1M 9AD

Australian Homoeopathic Association
c/o 16a Edward Street, Gordon, NSW 2027

International Foundation for Homoeopathy
2366 Eastlake East, No 301, Seattle, WA 98102, USA

Osteopathy

Many headaches are the result of problems in the neck and spine, and osteopathy is a type of treatment that has proved remarkably effective in dealing with these sorts of conditions. The joints in the neck are so close together that the slightest strain or damage to them can result in nerves being trapped, leading to muscular spasm. When the neck is put out of alignment, as well as producing headaches it can affect other parts of the body that depend on a balanced skeletal structure.

The osteopath will usually work from X-rays, and will manipulate the affected joints back into position. Sometimes the relief is instantaneous, but often it takes a while for the compressed nerve to recover. The manipulation may be quite forceful and is combined with massage techniques to relieve tension in muscle groups and other soft tissues. Osteopaths believe that this combination has a curative effect on the whole circulation as well as simply correcting the neck problem.

There are now stringent training requirements for anyone wishing to become a registered osteopath, and the ruling bodies insist on the highest standards of professional conduct. Some non-registered osteopaths have made extravagant claims concerning some of the conditions they can treat and this has led to the whole profession being viewed with scepticism. If, however, you choose a qualified practitioner obtained from one of the addresses below then it can be an excellent form of non-drug therapy for headaches caused by problems in the neck. As with most other forms of alternative treatment it is not available on the NHS in Britain and it is easy to quickly run up a sizeable bill. Again the general rule applies that a marked improvement should be felt within four appointments or else this line of therapy should be abandoned.

London School of Osteopathy
110 Richmond Road, Putney, London SW15

British and European Osteopathic Association
10 Sandringham Court, Dorset Road, Sutton, Surrey SM2 6NG

American Osteopathic Association and
Canadian Osteopathic Association
PO Bin 1050, Carmel, CA 93921

Australian Osteopathic Association
71 Collins Street, Melbourne, Victoria

Chiropractic

This technique bears a marked similarity to osteopathy, but is concerned solely with the joints in the body and not the surrounding soft tissue. It works on the theory that headaches are caused by misalignment of the joints of the neck, and the pain will disappear if this is corrected. The chiropractor uses a much gentler form of treatment than the osteopath as he softly eases the joints back into place. Generally this is totally painless, and patients are usually surprised by the click that is often heard and the sense of relief they feel. Sometimes some aching or tenderness may be experienced the following day as the bones settle down to their correct position. The treatment will be extended at the second session to a check of the alignment of bones in the rest of the body, working along the theory that a misplacement in one area may well cause a problem in another. All the skill lies in the hands and the correction is done by a gentle yet rapid springing motion. The pressure is no more than that of a light nudge to set the bone back into position. Chiropractic treats the whole person, which means examining all the joints of the body at each consultation as it is wrong to treat just the immediate area around the head and neck.

Addresses for registered chiropractors:

The British Chiropractic Association
Premier House, 10 Greycoat Place, London SW1P 1SB

The Institute of Pure Chiropractic
P.O. Box 126, Oxford OX2 8RH

American Chiropractic Association
1916 Wilson Blvd, Arlington, VA 22201

International Chiropractors Association
1901 L Street, N.W. Suite 800, Washington DC 20036

Hypnosis

This is one of the most powerful and effective methods of curing headaches, especially when you learn the technique of self-hypnosis which can be utilized at any time. Nobody fully understands the exact meaning of the state of hypnosis. Sceptics suggest it is similar to sleep, but this is certainly not true, as in sleep people are not conscious of where they are but a hypnotized person knows everything that is happening. Ideas and suggestions made during hypnosis can be resisted or utterly rejected.

Nobody can be hypnotized against their will, a point that is reassuring to many patients.

The hypnotic state actually lies somewhere between being awake and being asleep, where all the subject's protective reflexes are present. You will feel drowsy and relaxed but completely aware of what is happening around you. It is not dissimilar to the half-awake, half-asleep state you reach just before dropping off to sleep or when coming round in the morning. In other words it is an extremely pleasant state of awareness from which you would wake if any sudden emergency happened.

The hypnotherapist uses this relaxed level of consciousness to try to discover the root of the problem through regression, i.e. taking the client back to previous experiences, or by using subliminal suggestion to eradicate the problem. There are various methods for inducing hypnosis, and the ease of achieving this seems to depend upon the confidence and trust which the patient has in the therapist. Although the first session may take some time to overcome an initial resistance, once hypnosis is achieved then a simple method can be programmed into the person's mind so that on future appointments the hypnotic state can be reached quickly. Some therapists can do it by counting and in my own situation I achieve it by taking five deep breaths. It is worth stressing that no one can be hypnotized by someone coming into a room and saying a single word or phrase. This theory is simply for comedies on the television and bears no relation to reality.

It is possible to remember clearly events that have happened many years previously and often well back into childhood. These may be pleasant but usually the therapist is looking for troublesome situations that may have produced long-term harmful effects. If these are cleared from the subconscious mind they will cease to be a problem. Migraine in particular is related to past incidents that have unknowingly been stored away.

Just as important as going back in time are the auto-suggestions the therapist makes during the session. By introducing positive thoughts in to the subconscious mind they can clearly influence the way a person behaves in the future. Lack of confidence and fear of flying are two conditions that respond well.

In particular relation to headaches, it is usual to teach the patient the technique of self-hypnosis where you can put yourself into a hypnotic state at any time. The pure relaxation itself can relieve the pain but making positive suggestions as well — in other words telling the headache to go away — can reinforce the effect. Migraine and muscular headaches are the two conditions that respond particularly well to this technique. Surprisingly, the ability to hypnotize yourself can be learnt in a single session although it does take practice to achieve a deep state. Every time you experience a headache, by putting yourself 'under', you can obtain fast relief. A particular feature of self-hypnosis that I was taught by one therapist is to discover a place in my mind in which to escape when in need of relaxation. One of the most peaceful scenes I remember was on a sandy beach in North Wales on a beautiful summer's morning watching the sun rise over a calm sea. My therapist programmed my mind to take me back there whenever I practise self-hypnosis. This is very relaxing when carried out half-way through a busy Monday morning surgery! Waking from self-hypnosis is easy and is usually done by counting, or in my case, being disturbed by my next patient!

Confidence in and rapport with the therapist is very important, so care should be taken in selecting a suitable one. This is not always as easy as it seems, as there are now approximately 80 organizations in Britain from which to choose. Word of mouth is often the best way to find a specialist, but always rely on your own instincts as if you dislike the therapist on sight you will probably not benefit much from the treatment.

I have described hypnosis in some length as it is very effective in migraine and muscular headaches and the art of self-hypnosis is easy to learn. Everyone suffers from stress, so even if you do not suffer from either of these types of headache, hypnosis can be most beneficial in relieving the strains of modern life and as a consequent boost to the immune system.

To simplify the choice of therapists and to find a qualified practitioner in your area, look in your Yellow Pages. In Britain, you could also write to the following addresses:

The Association of Qualified Curative Hypnotherapists
10 Balaclava Road, Kings Heath, Birmingham.

The National Council of Psychotherapists
and Hypnotherapy Register
1 Clovelly Road, Ealing, London W5.

CHAPTER 12

To the future

Someday, no doubt, a pill will be produced that will cure all headaches, and for most people this would bring tremendous relief. Unfortunately it is probable that the medication will merely suppress the symptom of headache without in any way treating the underlying condition. In other words, it will only be a glorified painkiller and no one will really benefit. Pain is a vital protective mechanism within the body which, although unpleasant, prevents further damage to the affected part. If we accidentally touch something hot, then the pain makes us automatically take away our hand; and if we have a stomach ulcer we experience pain on eating fatty food, alerting us to change to a diet containing less fat with a subsequent reduction in the harmful acid level. Headaches work in the same way to warn us that all is not well and therefore it is insufficient to take the Western road to therapy consisting of simple analgesia. However some people's severity of headache seems far in excess of a simple warning and indeed recent developments suggest that there may be an underlying defect in a certain part of the brain.

In the surgery I am often asked why some people seem far more sensitive to pain and develop headaches more often than others. Whilst this undoubtedly is related to the condition of their immune system, recent research has shown that there may be other factors. There are special nerves in the body that are responsible for feeling pain, and these send a message to the brain which then interprets the signal and the pain is felt. Up to that point, the pain has been going on outside our consciousness. This explains why if you bang your toe there is a slight delay in feeling the pain whilst the message passes up to the brain, even though you know it is going to hurt! On the way to the brain, the painful impulses have to pass through an area called the brain stem which lies between the top of the neck and the base of the brain itself. Everyone has a brain stem and it is responsible for functions like breathing and blood pressure control. In actual fact it has dozens of separate functions but the one that concerns us most is that it contains a system which is responsible for deciding what sort of nervous impulses actually reach the brain.

If you are at a noisy party, for example, it is often difficult to hear what people are saying but if you become involved in a conversation with someone of interest then your brain will actually exclude much of the surrounding noise. The brain stem is responsible then for deciding which things from the outside world are going to be allowed through to your conscious mind. There is now an indication that in the brain stem there is a kind of gate which only allows pain signals to pass through when it is open. This is why sometimes 'in the heat of battle', pain is not felt until much later. Sportsmen and women have been known to break bones and not feel the pain until they relax in the changing room after the match.

The brain stem normally works in such a way that only the things which are liable to damage the body actually cause you to feel pain. This is certainly the case with headaches, and it should result in some corrective action. However, there is no doubt that sometimes this mechanism goes over the top and the warning pain is far too intense. In headaches, it seems, the primary difference between each of us is the way the brain stem allows the painful information to pass to the brain. It has recently been discovered that people who are prone to headaches have a low resistance to all types of pain and not just for headaches. In a series of experiments designed to measure their appreciation of pain, regular headache sufferers found sounds uncomfortable and then painful much sooner than those who had never had headaches. Every migraine sufferer will tell you that during an attack all lights seem brighter and sounds appear louder than they do normally.

It would seem possible, therefore, that people who experience headaches that far exceed a simple warning may in fact have an abnormality of the brain stem. It is interesting that during an attack of migraine the headache often pounds in time with the pulse. In the same area as the pain gate are the parts of the brain stem which are involved in the control of blood flow in and around the brain. One of the chemicals involved in this flow is called serotonin and this has also been shown to have an effect on pain. It seems to dampen down the flow of nervous impulses that pass through the gate into the brain. Serotonin has many actions throughout the body but its role in pain appears particularly crucial in headaches.

If the level of serotonin is low in the body, then pain is felt much more easily. Thus, if there is a degree of chemical imbalance within the brain stem it may lead to a lowering of the serotonin level with a subsequent increase in pain sensation and the development of headache. This can explain why cheese, chocolate, and red wine can produce muscular and migraine headaches, as they all contain an ingredient which interferes with the chemical balance of the brain stem. Hormones and stress lead to similar chemical changes. One day in the not too distant future, the exact nature of this imbalance of serotonin will be discovered and the exaggerated response of some people to headaches will be relieved. However, even then it will not reduce the frequency of the headaches, merely the intensity, so it will still be necessary to look at the reasons for them.

The final relief of headaches will ultimately rest in our own hands. Everyone suffers with headaches to some degree and this is partly because of the high-pressure life that we all lead. Even if our individual stress levels are low, there are still too many demands made on us and precious little time to be ourselves. We do not have a moment in the day to stop and think, let alone the time to be quiet to work out the root cause of our headaches. Long gone are the peace and stillness of the winter evenings when the fire burned in the grate, the lamps were lit and the room was bathed in a warm glow. There was a calmness about those times where one could gather thoughts together and gain strength to deal with life's problems. Now it is all television, gas fires, telephone calls, even trips to the local supermarket at 9 o'clock at night, and nowhere is there space in the day to recharge ourselves.

We all want to be healthier, and many times we promise to make changes in our lifestyle. We all intend to give up chocolate and cakes to lose that spare tyre around the waist, to take an early morning run, and to relax more often. However, it is always starting tomorrow and tomorrow never seems to come, so we remain stressed and at risk of illness. Changing to a healthy lifestyle takes energy, effort and most of all willpower. Whilst other people can give encouragement, it is down to ourselves to instigate the necessary changes.

By following the steps outlined in this book, it should now be possible for everyone with headaches to identify the cause and take the appropriate actions to remedy them. In some cases this will be easy whereas others may find it takes a major adaptation in lifestyle. This usually means certain sacrifices and strong willpower but the rewards in the end are well worth it. Not only does it mean the end of the troublesome headaches but your health in general will improve, especially if you have taken the recommended steps to boost your immune system. I cannot emphasize enough the importance of your own natural defence mechanism in fighting off illness. At some times in this book it has been necessary to advise seeking professional help, but this has been kept to a minimum and I have discussed drugs very little as they play no real part in the management of headaches.

We are living in an interesting time for health care, where conventional doctors in the Western world are at long last starting to recognize the benefits of alternative therapy. An increasing number of general practitioners are using one or more of these methods to treat patients in their surgeries. It is not uncommon now to find acupuncture and homoeopathy featuring quite prominently in a GP's repertoire. The latter is now available on the health service in Britain and hopefully this will soon extend into other complementary therapies. Certainly for the headache sufferer it is excellent news, as it means the doctor will treat them as a whole person and not just as a symptom.

Do not let headaches master you and drive you to despair. They can be relieved so they play no part in your day-to-day living and do not affect the quality of life. You were born to be happy and healthy and you owe it to yourself to achieve this goal. Use this book to enable you to do just that.

Index